One in Eight

A Breast Cancer Journey

Practical Guide for Patients, Families, and Workplaces

VIKKI ESPINOSA

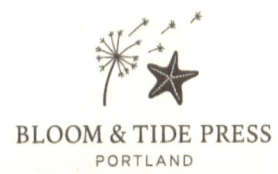

BLOOM & TIDE PRESS

PORTLAND

One in Eight: A Breast Cancer Journey and Practical Guide for Patients, Families, and Workplaces

For permissions, contact the publisher at:
press@bloomandtidepress.com

Published by Bloom & Tide Press
ISBN: 979-8-9939050-0-6
Printed in the United States of America

Personal Experience Clause – The content of this book is based on the author's personal experiences with breast cancer treatment and recovery. Every individual's medical situation is unique, and treatment outcomes vary. The author's experiences should not be interpreted as universal or predictive of any other individual's medical path.

Emotional and Psychological Disclaimer – This book contains discussions of cancer treatment, personal loss, and emotional challenges. While the intent is to provide guidance and support, some content may be triggering for certain individuals. If you are struggling emotionally, please consider seeking support from a licensed therapist, counselor, or trusted support network. You are not alone, and help is available.

No Liability Statement – The author and publisher disclaim any liability for the use or misuse of the information contained in this book. The content is based on personal experiences and research. Still, it should not be relied upon as a substitute for professional advice. Every reader's journey is unique, and treatment outcomes vary.

Editing and Design Credits

Cover Design: Sarah Moyle
Author Photo by: Talli Koppel
Edited by: Stephanie Baturoni

For additional resources, updates, or to connect with the author, visit: vikkiespinosawrites.com

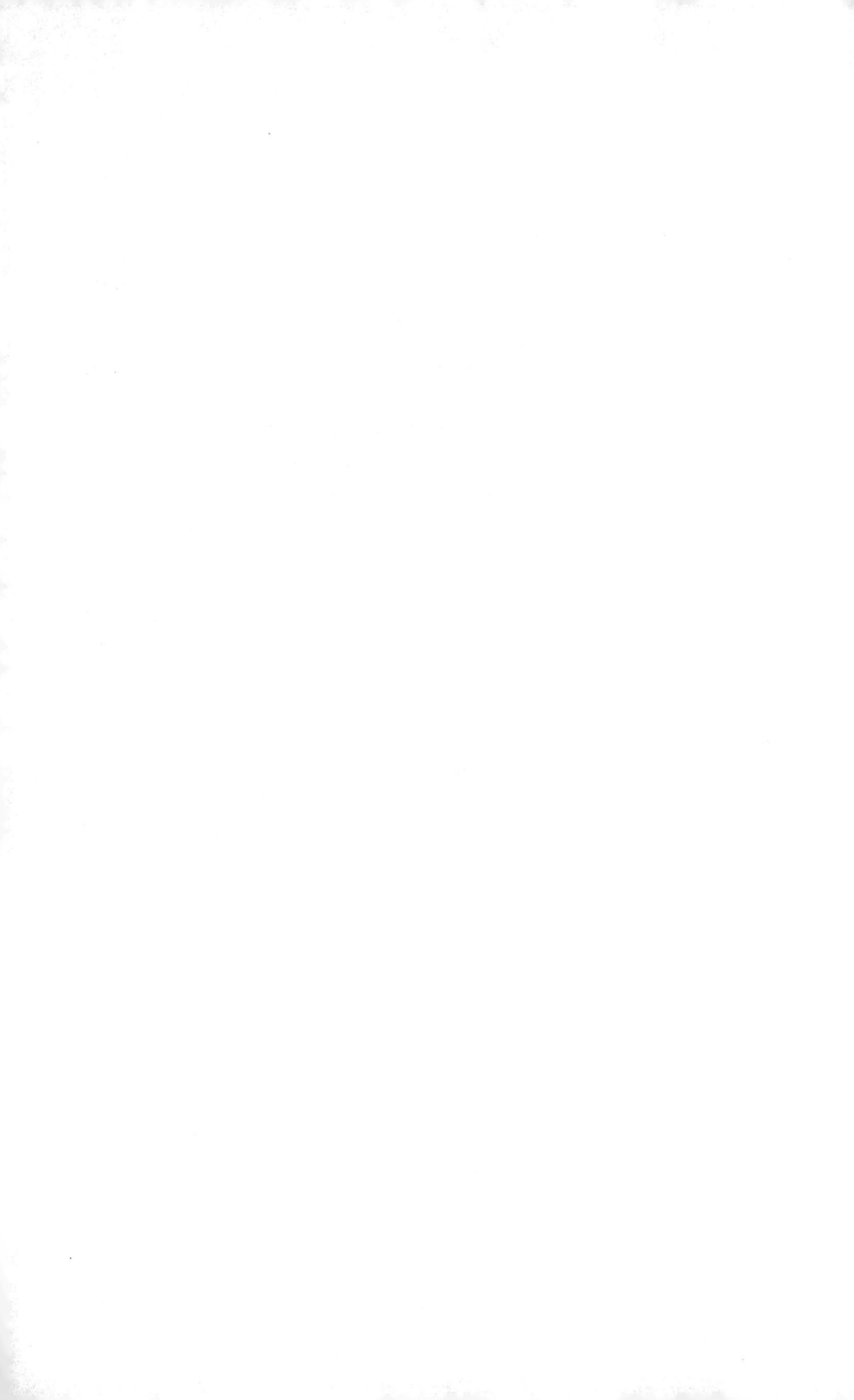

Editing and Design Credits

Cover Design: Sarah Moyle
Author Photo by: Talli Koppel
Edited by: Stephanie Baturoni

For additional resources, updates, or to connect with the author, visit: vikkiespinosawrites.com

Dedication

I dedicate this book to my husband and partner of 40 years, Gus. 2023 tested him in ways I'll never forget. I was not the only person he had to support through medical issues. He managed it all with his steadfast support for all of us while doing his job. I could not have been as strong without his wise words and unwavering support.

Gus, you are the love of my life. My rock. My best friend. My foundation. I adore you.

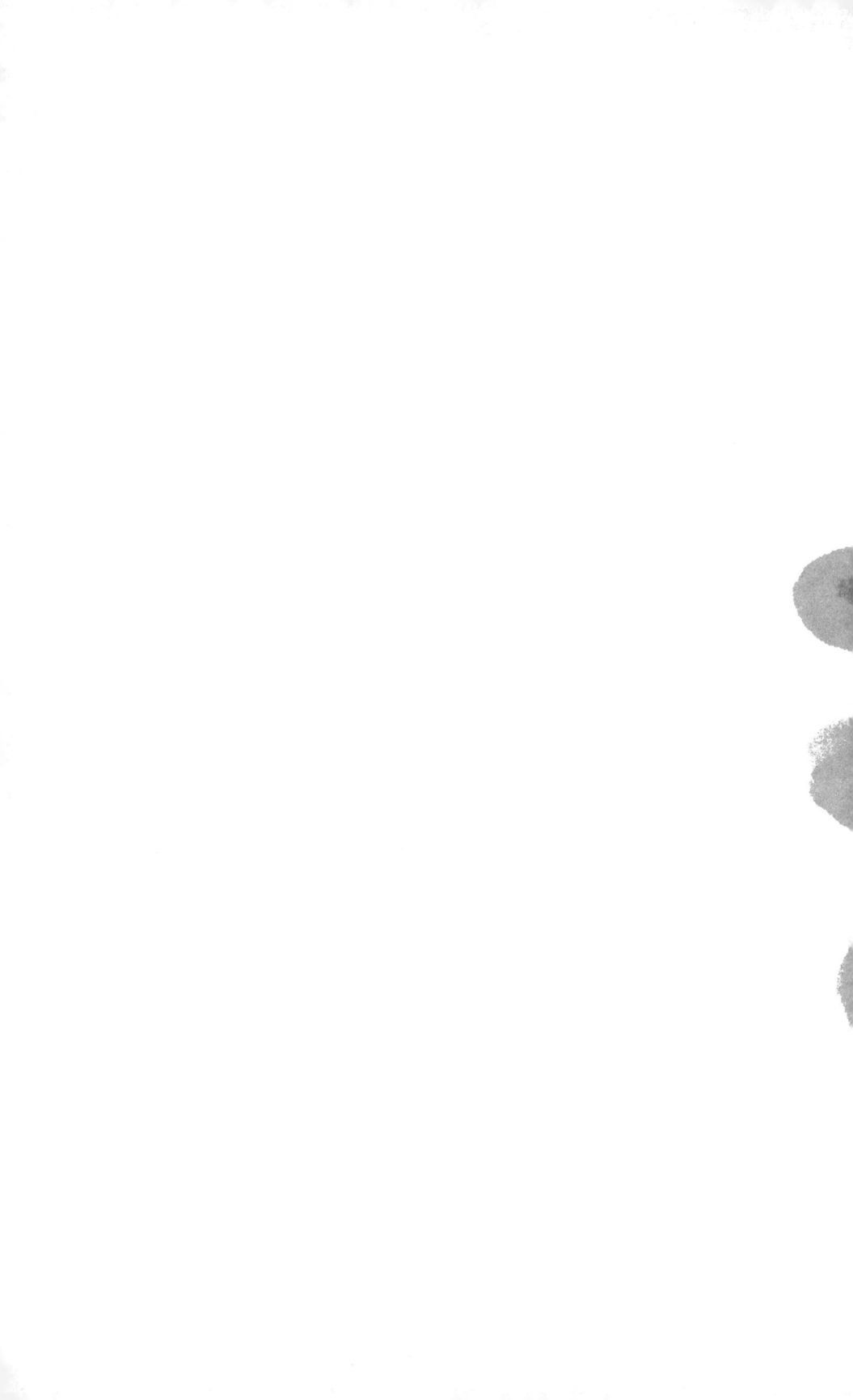

Cancer took so much from me. But in what was left, I found the parts of myself that could never be taken—my humor, my stubbornness, and the quiet will to keep moving forward. This is the story of what I lost, and everything I found along the way.

— Vikki Espinosa

CONTENTS

How to Use This Book

If you're newly diagnosed or in active treatment, you may want to begin with **Section One: The Journey**. This is my story—what happened, how it felt, what surprised me, and what I wish I'd known. Sometimes reading someone else's experience makes the path ahead feel less overwhelming.

If you're living in the space after treatment, you might start with **Section Two: Life After Treatment**. These chapters dig into identity, grief, resilience, and rebuilding your life when you're no longer in survival mode but don't quite feel "back to normal."

If you're looking for community, shared wisdom, or just reassurance that there's no single "right" way to navigate cancer, turn to **Section Three: Other Voices**. These stories broaden the lens and remind you that every journey is different—and valid.

If you're a caregiver, partner, friend, or neighbor, head to **Section Four: A Guide for Patients and Caregivers**. This section is practical and direct: what to say, what not to say, how to support someone without overstepping, and how to understand the emotional landscape of cancer from the outside.

If you're a manager, HR leader, or colleague, **Section Five: A Guide for Workplaces and Managers** offers guidance for supporting employees through diagnosis, treatment, and return-to-work transitions. Cancer shows up at work whether we plan for it or not.

If you're preparing for treatment or want tools to stay organized and informed, explore **Section Six: Getting Ready**. It includes planning lists, questions to ask your doctor, strategies for daily life, and a collection of practical resources to help you move forward.

If you process through writing or reflection, **Section Seven** is your space. You'll find journaling practices and final reflections to help you make sense of everything you're carrying.

Section Eight includes gratitude, resources, book club questions, and the people (and dogs) who helped carry me through. It's a place to linger if you want community, recommendations, or a softer landing at the end.

So read straight through or skip to the parts you need right now. Fold down pages, highlight passages, scribble notes in the margins, and share sections with the people who would benefit from this information. My hope is that this book will feel less like a lecture and more like a companion, something you can return to when you need practical help, honest reflection, or just a reminder that you don't have to face this alone.

Introduction:
The Day Everything Changed

On February 9, 2023, the sun peeked through the clouds in Portland, Oregon. I snapped a photo in the hospital waiting room and sent it to my family to let them know I was waiting for my mammogram. I wanted to believe everything was fine—that whatever I had been feeling was exaggerated or just a misunderstanding. But somewhere deep in the back of my mind, a quiet voice was preparing me for the worst.

That photo marks my last cancer-free moment.

After an anomaly showed up on my mammogram, I was diagnosed with Stage 1 DCIS (ductal carcinoma in situ), triple-positive breast cancer. The second mammogram and ultrasound confirmed it. My doctor performed a biopsy right then and there. Before the official results even came back, she looked at me and said she was 99% confident I had breast cancer.

One in eight women will be diagnosed with breast cancer. Think of eight coworkers, friends, or family members. Statistically, one of them will face this diagnosis. Women are also being diagnosed younger—some in their 20s or 30s—often before they've even thought about mammograms. It feels terrifying. It feels unfair.

What I Wish I Had Known Before Diagnosis

- Take a deep breath. You don't have to process everything today.

- Ask for help. You will need it, even if you don't want to admit it.

- Your body will change. Some of the changes will be temporary, some won't. Even if you don't feel like yourself for a while, you're not lost or erased. You are still here. It may take time to recognize yourself in your new form.

- There is no right way to do this. You don't have to be "strong" all the time. You don't have to be positive every day.

- It will take longer than you think. Recovery doesn't end when treatment does—and it may look different than you imagined. But healing is still possible.

What about You?

I've had two years of post-treatment mammograms. They were clear. Fortunately, I got the "all clear" right after my scans, without having to wait for bad news. Those moments were full of relief, gratitude, and cautious optimism.

What about you?

When was your last mammogram?

Do you know your family history? Mine doesn't include the BRCA gene, but that didn't mean I was immune to breast cancer.

Are you doing monthly self-exams?

When was your mom's last mammogram? Your sister's? Your daughter's? Your wife's?

Ask. And if it's been more than a year since that woman's last exam—or yours—schedule one immediately.

I've met so many women who wish they had done it sooner. Some got out of the habit during COVID. Others were too busy with work, with kids, and with life. Some thought they were safe because no one in their family had been diagnosed.

Years of learning and teaching resilience training have taught me this: **you can't pour from an empty cup.** You have to take care of yourself before you can care for anyone else. Scheduling that mammogram isn't just for you. It's for the people who love you.

This book is my way of giving back. Whether you're the patient, the caregiver, or someone who loves or cares for them, I hope reading about my journey makes yours a little easier.

Fondly,
Vikki

Key People

Before we dive into my diary and the subsequent essays and information on how to help others with a cancer diagnosis, I want to introduce you to my friends, family, and medical team. These are the people who love me, support me, and help me through. I have also included all the dogs' names at the end of the book. Dogs are magic.

Gus – my husband of 30 years. We met when I was seventeen, and he was twenty. He would like you to think it's the other way around – that he's the younger one. He's an engineer who works on computer hardware and software architecture, designing safety and reliability features in technology that enhance lives.

Julia – our eldest daughter. She is twenty-five. She has a lovely little cat named Minerva and works nearby. She loves music, coffee, cats, and books.

Claire – our youngest daughter. She is twenty-two. She also lives, studies, and works nearby. She has two cats, Juno and Venus. She loves cats, good food, and exploring the world.

Erin H – a mom friend. Our oldest daughters did sports together. Erin battled breast cancer some years ago and was amazingly supportive and helpful during the period when I didn't know what I didn't know. You'll read some of her story.

Talli is a dear friend I met at work. We have known each other for almost 30 years. She lives six minutes away and was the person who checked in and supported me the most during treatment. Her short texts made me feel remembered, cared for, and encouraged as I faced each new challenge. She loves to take pictures of birds and wildlife – and occasionally people. (She took my photo.)

Sarah – my creative and talented former work-wife. We worked together for many years and have remained close after my retirement. She approaches life with curiosity and wonder. She can do all sorts of things, from cutting hair to illustrating and designing book covers (like this one!) to teaching people how to be creative. She is a fantastic mom to three wonderful kids. She is also the bonus mom for two other lovely children. You can check out her art and creative pursuits at **sarahmoyle.com**.

SECTION ONE

The Journey

Cancer doesn't enter life quietly—it shatters the rhythm of ordinary days. This section is my story as it unfolded: the phone calls, the treatments, the private moments of fear and unexpected flashes of humor. It's the truth of what it felt like to be diagnosed and to keep moving through.

Chapter 1: "You Have Cancer"

When I retired from Intel, I thought I had a clean runway ahead of me: time to build my consulting practice, a few paid talks already booked, the freedom to finally design my own calendar. My annual mammogram was scheduled for the week after my last day. Nine days after my retirement date, I was diagnosed with breast cancer.

It stopped everything. The momentum I'd been building, the excitement, the plans—I didn't know how to hit pause, but suddenly I had no choice.

After decades spent guiding other people through their hardest seasons, I was the one in unfamiliar territory. Vulnerable. Needing help. Completely outside the identity I'd spent years strengthening. It felt foreign and uncomfortable, like stepping into a life I hadn't agreed to.

Deciding Who to Tell (and how)

After my diagnosis, I struggled with deciding who to tell. I didn't want to deal with the wave of empathy—or worse, pity—that might result from sharing the news with too many people. I also wasn't sure I could handle others' emotions.

I've always been the advisor, the counselor, the one everyone confides in. While most of it is under the guise of career development, many people have shared intimate details of their lives with me so I could help guide them forward. I knew I couldn't handle being on the other side of those conversations, so, in agreement with my closest friends and family, we kept the circle small.

To keep others updated, I started a blog in a private Facebook group. It allowed me to share what was happening and receive encouragement from those I trusted most.

After reading so many other women's stories on Reddit, I realized I was lucky. I didn't encounter anyone who said anything hurtful or upsetting. I chose the right people, and they were wonderful. The most important thing they did was to provide support without asking me to manage their feelings about my diagnosis.

Receiving calls from the supermarket to ask if I needed anything, or having soup or dinner dropped off after chemo, was incredibly helpful. They never did anything without asking first, and I'm deeply grateful for their love and support.

I did not want to explain everything repeatedly, so using a Facebook group allowed me to write entries they could read and respond to at their own pace. Their reactions made me feel connected. It felt good to document everything and get it out, without listening to others for their feelings or concerns. I knew some other friends would want to debate the treatment path my medical team had chosen, and others would want to share their fears and worries. I didn't have the energy or mental capacity to listen to everyone who might know about my cancer. Also, seeing how far I had come and how much longer I had to go was therapeutic and helpful. I tracked the number of treatments and the percentage of completed treatments obsessively.

I recommend journaling; however it works for you. One of my friends who was diagnosed after me kept a video journal and posted regularly so her circle would know where she was in the process and what she was feeling and needing.

I discuss journaling as a healing tool in Chapter 37.

The following chapters include direct excerpts from my journal and Facebook group messages. This section of the book is deeply personal—a raw glimpse into my thoughts, fears, and triumphs as I navigated my breast cancer diagnosis and treatment. These entries aren't polished essays but snapshots of real-time moments, reflecting the rollercoaster of emotions and challenges I faced.

I chose to include them because I want readers to see what it's like, unfiltered. Whether you're going through something similar, supporting a loved one, or simply seeking to understand, I hope these words remind you that you are not alone.

Day 1: Failed Mammogram

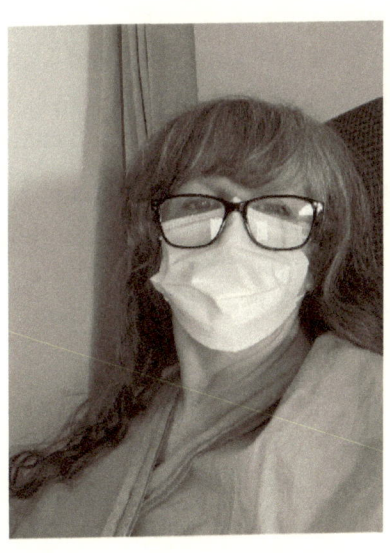

In January of 2023, while I was finishing my career at Intel and preparing for retirement, I scheduled my regular mammogram. A meeting came up, so I rescheduled it for February, which was why it was a week after my retirement date.

Gus and our eldest daughter, Julia, were in Florida visiting my mother-in-law, Raquel, who still doesn't know about my cancer. Given her age and health, we decided to shield her from stress and worry.

On February 7, at St. Vincent's Hospital, I had my first mammogram of the year. When they reviewed the results, they told me that I needed follow-up imaging at the Good Samaritan Breast Clinic in downtown Portland, Oregon. They scheduled me for February 9, giving themselves 90 minutes to perform high-resolution mammograms, ultrasounds, and, if needed, a biopsy.

I wasn't too worried—this had happened before, and it had turned out to be a benign cyst. Still, I appreciated the staff's thoroughness.

Day 3: You Have Cancer

I sat in the sun for a few minutes on the roof of the parking garage and snapped a photo, thinking it was nice how warm it was, and briefly wondered if this would be a life-altering visit. Then I went in, and they got me ready. At Good Sam, you sit in a little waiting room with a rocking chair, and each technician comes for you. After changing into a gown, I snapped a second photo and sent it to our family group chat.

The first to get me out of my room was the mammogram technician. She was lovely, and the machine was gentler than the one I'd experienced previously. 3D is definitely easier on the squeeze. We finished, and she led me back into my little waiting room.

Then, the ultrasound tech came for me. She brought me into a long, wide room. I thought that was weird since, when you get a scan, most ultrasound rooms are dark and small. (I've had more ultrasounds than I can count due to other illnesses and injuries.) I was still in my gown from the previous test. She got me on the table, shoved a wedge under my left shoulder, and got to work after applying the gel. After taking pictures and measuring the size of something in my left breast, she spent a lot of time in my armpit (presumably checking the lymph nodes). She finished, covered me with a towel, and asked me to wait while she spoke with the radiologist.

The radiologist came in a few minutes later. The first thing out of her mouth was, "I am 99% sure you have cancer." At least, that is the first thing I remember hearing. I am a big proponent of getting the bad news out fast, and she certainly delivered. She also grabbed my shoulder and said, "This is why we do routine screens. We caught it early. It is small. While you are here and ready, I'd like to do a biopsy."

I agreed with her plan and signed some paperwork. Then she told me I would be numbed, and she'd use the ultrasound to guide a gun-like instrument into my breast to remove two pieces of tissue. She would then use the same instrument to leave behind a marker – a Savi Scout so anyone looking could easily find the tumor again. She said, "The gun is loud, so don't flinch when it goes off." She set it off several times before she started, so I would know what to expect.

As the radiologist left the room to prepare for the procedure, I cried. There were no sobs, no heaving chest, just tears leaking out and down my face as I realized I was alone in that room and facing the unknown.

She returned with the tech and two carts covered in instruments and supplies. The reason the room was so wide and had so much space was revealed. They needed the room for the carts.

The numbing needle went in; it was not too bad. Then the radiologist pushed in deeper and deadened my entire left breast. I thought, "So far, it's not bad, definitely not as bad as Novocain at the dentist or when the podiatrist numbed my big toe to remove an ingrown nail."

The next thing I knew, she was telling me she was ready to pull the trigger on her biopsy gun. She took two samples and then told me she was placing the Savi Scout. I got a simple

Band-Aid on my breast, then she told me to wipe off any residual gel, wrap up, and return to the room to wait for another set of mammogram scans. She described it as an easy squeeze to ensure they knew where the Scout was.

After the scans, nurses sat with me. They reviewed a notebook containing information and a lengthy list of upcoming appointments. They didn't ask me if the times worked for my schedule. They just scheduled everything and assumed I would prioritize accordingly. After all, it was time to put myself first.

Then I went home. To wait. For pathology to confirm what the radiologist was 99% sure I had. I knew Julia and Gus were on the plane to come home, and I wanted them to have time to process my news before landing, since I needed to pick them up from the airport later that evening. I let them know while they were traveling. I am not sure they will ever forgive me for delivering the news this way. However, I knew I couldn't pick them up at the airport and keep myself together for the drive home unless they already knew.

I managed to put my thoughts aside for most of the afternoon, then met them at the airport. Then we waited for news on Monday, when I was due to hear from the doctor. I decided not to tell anyone else since I did not have 100% clarity on the diagnosis or what was next. I was in shock and some denial.

I did know what appointments were coming, though. The breast surgeon, the medical (chemo) oncologist, a genealogist, an MRI scan, and some blood work. We got confirmation on February 13 that I did indeed have breast cancer. They were not sure about the HER2/neu number, so they sent some of my tissue sample for a FISH test. [1]

More waiting. And then the answer.

Officially, I was Stage 1. Estrogen+2, Progesterone +1, HER2/neu +2, Fish Positive, MIB (replication rate) high at 60/70%. The mass was at 2 o'clock on the left side, 1.7 CM. It was the size of a pencil eraser. And it was going to try to kill me.

After some extra research and debate, I was put on a cocktail of three drugs for chemo—Taxol *(a brand name for paclitaxel)*, Perjeta, and Herceptin. Sessions one, four, seven, and twelve would include all three drugs. The rest are Taxol only. They say I will lose my hair.

Day 5: Meds: This is Only the Beginning

So far, symptoms have been nerve pain in the back of my legs, diarrhea, nausea, exhaustion, and bad facial acne that requires steroids.

I have gone to two therapy sessions to help me deal with the loss of physicality and the perceived loss of control over my life. I have one more to go, and the therapist has been excellent, with good tactical suggestions and books to help me figure this out. The one that helped the most was *When Life Hits Hard: How to Transcend Grief, Crisis, and Loss* by Russ Harris.

---

[1] HER2/neu is a protein that can promote the growth of cancer cells. In about 1 in 5 breast cancers, the cells make an excess of this protein due to a gene mutation, which makes the cancer more aggressive. Doctors test tumors for HER2 status to determine the best course of treatment. One way to test for this is the FISH test (Fluorescence In Situ Hybridization), which looks for extra copies of the HER2 gene in the cancer cells. It's considered more precise than other tests, and the results help determine whether drugs like Herceptin (trastuzumab) might be effective.

I have discovered VR workouts and have been having fun with my friends, Talli and Sarah, playing mini golf. I have felt amazing support and care from friends and neighbors. I am doing okay today and going to lunch with Julia. My biggest thing is trying to feel normal, and like my life did not stop with my diagnosis. I appreciate the invitations to dinners, activities, and visits more than you all know. Little memes in a text message, funny TikToks, things to read, and TED Talks to watch are all greatly appreciated.

I have a few things lined up for my small consulting business: a "How Women Rise" workshop, a panel appearance (paid), and potentially a contract with a big company to deliver Job Crafting workshops. I am taking it slowly since I do not know if my energy will continue to wax and wane or if I'll get increasingly tired as this goes along.

Day 15: Asking for Support

Hi! I want all of you to be aware of what's happening, and I wanted a place to talk about it all at once, so I don't have to repeat myself. The most significant gift you can give me is the gift of normality.

Tell me what is going on, go to lunch with me, or let's all eat dinner together. I don't want to dwell on what is happening to me or only talk about cancer and my treatment plan.

You are welcome to ask as many questions as you like here. They will help me with my questions for the medical professionals.

Update: I will have minor surgery on Monday to get a medicine port put in my upper chest. I will have it for a year. Check in at 2:30 pm. Surgery is at 4:00 pm. I should be home by 6:00 pm. Everything is at Good Sam Hospital downtown on NW 22nd.

This week, I have an MRI and an echocardiogram.

Next week is medical oncology, to learn about the drugs and chemo I will be taking.

The week after is the first visit with the plastic surgeon. Surgery should be done sometime in August. They want me to do all the drugs and treatment first to make sure it is working before they remove the tumor. It is small. 1.7 cm x 1 cm x 1 cm. They hope to shrink it or kill it with the therapy.

Day 21: Port Placement

Today started with a bit of fun—chasing our dog, Dakota, down to get a urine sample. He has a doctor's appointment this morning to see how his organs are responding to the food I make for him. Before I started cooking for him, his pancreas and kidney levels were not good. They do a senior dog blood and urine panel to check on things. Since we stopped the medicated eye drops (the groomer nicked his eye last week), he has been doing much better. The eye drops were taxing his heart, based on the contraindications listed on the paper that came with the bottle. It has been quite a week caring for the old dude. He is good this morning. He will be mad in about an hour when we visit the vet. Good distraction since I cannot eat all day. Gus will drop me off at the hospital at 2:30 pm; the procedure is at 4 pm. And I should be ready to come home at six pm. I usually come out of anesthesia without too much trouble. I suppose four knee surgeries have helped prep me for today.

Day 23: Medical Oncology

My medical Oncology appointment is this morning. I find out my chemo schedule. And whatever else the doctors are going to give me. My IV pricks are healing well. They had to do two. The first one didn't work, but the one on the top of my hand did. Gus removed the heart-shaped dressing from my port this morning, so I could shower. I have a layer of tape underneath and then Steri-Strips. The incisions are pretty small. I cannot see the port opening under the tape. I have some bruising, and my chest is stiff, like when you overwork your pecs at the gym.[2]

Wendy came for lunch yesterday. Good to talk about our combined mobility issues and eat soup. She brought chocolate, and that always makes me feel better.

I will check in after the doctor today and record what is next.

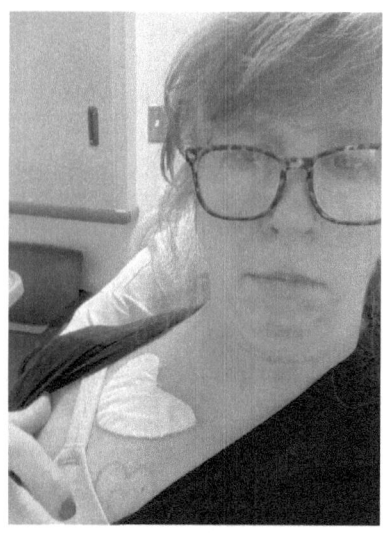

Update: Today was a rough day—two and a half hours at medical oncology. I learned I am Stage One.

That was good. It could also cause an insurance issue because what they want to do is give me the chemo first and then do surgery. That is not the current protocol for stage one patients. Usually, they do surgery first and then the drugs. Both the breast surgeon and the oncologist want to try the drugs first and surgery second. They submitted their plan to the insurance company, and now we have to wait to see if the insurance approves the doctors' plan. If the plan is approved, my first chemo treatment will be on March 10. If the insurance does not approve the change in the order of operations, they will instead do surgery first.

---

[2] I found out later that the port is entirely beneath the skin. You still get pricked, and the skin is sensitive. However, the needle then sits in the port, and it's a bigger opening than a vein, so that they can access it quickly and easily every time.

Yesterday, I had acupuncture for the horrific anesthesia hangover from the port insertion procedure. Colleen (my acupuncturist) got rid of the headache by needling between my toes, and I feel much better today. Mentally, I'm struggling a bit, but I am grateful for Anu's visit this evening. The surgery site is still tender. I am hoping it starts to let up tomorrow. Continuing to ice. The next thing is my rescheduled MRI on Saturday morning. I will see the plastic surgeon on Monday and get my baseline echocardiogram on Tuesday. And if we get approval from the insurance company, I will start chemo next Friday. They also discussed a bone density test at some point.

Day 27: Breast MRI

Yesterday morning, I had an MRI of both breasts. On my stomach with my boobs hanging free for 30 minutes, with an injection of contrast towards the end. Contrast makes you feel like you peed yourself. You feel all warm and weird as it moves around your body. Not pleasant. I still feel like a human pin cushion. It took two tries to get the IV in. The second guy knew what he was doing. They couldn't use my port because no one in the imaging department was trained to do so.

Late last night, the report came through with the results. Nothing weird in the right boob. The tumor had been sized correctly on the left via mammogram and ultrasound. And no other issues were noted. So, no surprises, which is perfect. And a relief.

Tomorrow, I will meet with the plastic surgeon. On Tuesday, I get my baseline echocardiogram. Nothing planned for Wednesday or Thursday. I will probably get a manicure and pedicure.

Friday is the first chemo. Gus is going with me. Then it is weekly on Thursdays at Good Sam's Cancer Center.

Let me know if anyone would like to drive and sit with me to relieve Gus.

Chapter 2: Treatment – Entering the Unknown

I had done everything I could to prepare. I had a cooler for the gloves and socks I would wear, along with the ice packs you tuck inside to prevent neuropathy.

I had snacks. Talli had given me a blanket. I had noise-canceling headphones and a small cross-stitch project (which I never completed). I had read about side effects and prepared a plan for every "what if," so I was telling myself I was ready.

But nothing really prepares you for sitting in that chair for the first time. The nurses wear extra personal protective equipment—gowns, gloves, and masks—when it's time to hook up the chemo to protect themselves. They double-check the drugs, and suddenly - it's happening. It's running into the IV and into your body. No protective gear is needed for the patient.

There's a difference between knowing what's coming and feeling it in your veins.

Day 31: The Day before Chemo

My bag is packed for tomorrow. Thanks to the Herreras for watching Dakota and dealing with his bathroom visits every two hours.

I still want to flee. But I know it is time to stand and fight. I have meds for nausea and diarrhea. I put a freezer in the bedroom for cold packs and popsicles. I also packed a kit for Gus's car in case I get sick on the way home.

My electronics are charged, and I have a spare power bank. Snacks, gum, and mints. My blanket from Talli. Cold gloves and socks will hopefully prevent neuropathy. I'm going to dress in layers. I already cut over a foot of my hair off. Sarah says she will come and cut more next week.

If you're preparing for chemo, see Section Four: Resources and Checklists for a list of what to bring and how to prepare.

I also got a notification that the wigs I ordered have been shipped.

Now, I need to pop a pill and see if I can sleep.

Day 33: After Chemo #1

The first chemo is done. It was a long day. Three drugs. They dripped slowly, with 30 minutes in between. There was no major reaction. The nurse—Emma—was great. I slept through most of it, wrapped in a blanket and wearing noise-canceling headphones blasting music. Poor Gus was bored senseless and forgot his earplugs.

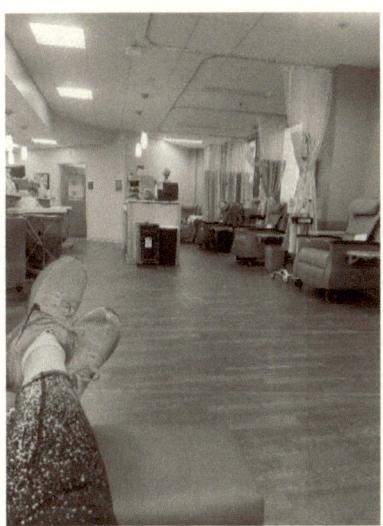

The infusion room is easy to clean, but that makes it rather barren. There is almost constant beeping as the infusion machines finish pumping meds into patients, and attention is needed from the nurses to make them stop their unrelenting noise. Nurses are constantly moving around, responding to alarms, unkinking lines, programming machines, donning protective gowns, and administering medications. Sometimes you have one bag of drugs and a flush of saline: other times, it's three drugs and other medications to counteract the side effects, and then the flushes to get every bit of the medication into you. Nurses change out the drugs until you've had them all, and finally remove the IV from your drug port and send you home with a band-aid.

I came home, ate dinner, watched TV, and snoozed on the couch.

My big mistake was lying flat in bed. I ended up with reflux and heartburn, a coughing fit, and feeling like I needed to throw up. I moved to the recliner in our room, so my head would be higher than my stomach. After taking some

Tylenol, Pepto, and water, I was able to settle down and get some sleep. I still have a headache and some mild heartburn—I managed not to vomit, though.

Sitting on the couch. I'm going to try to take a short walk and shower today.

F*ck Cancer.

Day 35: Aftermath

Spent most of yesterday sleeping. I had a nice visit from Erin H, who brought me things I didn't know I needed. These included wooden utensils, since metal ones may taste unpleasant at times. And a rubber-mat bottle opener for when I get so weak I can't open a jar. She says I'll lose my grip strength over time.

Talli and I played VR mini golf. I am getting better at not whacking the ball out of bounds.

I managed to make dinner for Gus while he went to pick up groceries for Julia, who has been under the weather.

Today, I see the psychologist. I need some coping skills to handle the lack of control I feel over this whole process.

The next chemo is on Thursday. I'll be having acupuncture beforehand, to boost my white cell count, and afterward to deal with the headache that I can't seem to shake.

The first treatment was behind me, but I didn't know yet how my body would react. The side effects started creeping in sooner than expected.

Day 36: Midnight Cramps

Last night was the worst of this journey so far. After I got back from therapy, I had leg cramps most of yesterday afternoon. Gus got me a long heating pad, and that helped some. Julia did some internet searching and recommended I drink electrolytes and eat an orange for some natural sugar. I managed to get into bed and onto the heating pad. My glutes and hamstrings were contracted and painful. I woke up at 2 am, writhing in pain. It felt like I was made like monkey bread[3]—all stuck together—and something was trying to pull me apart. I tried moving around. More heat. Massage from Gus. It was awful. Could not sit still. Could not relax. This is certainly not for the faint of heart. I took an Xanax and then some ibuprofen. We added a cold pack to my chest while my leg and butt were on the heating pad. Finally, the cramping began to subside. I fell asleep after talking to the doctor, who was unable to provide any helpful advice; there was no way I was braving a ride to the ER. I will need to figure out what to do next time. That was unbearable.

I got some sleep, and today I am sore. It's like I worked out too hard. I had some breakfast and tea. I'm hoping to take a walk and get some light exercise to see if I can lessen the muscle aches.

F*ck Cancer and chemo. You think you're doing okay, but you're actually getting progressively worse. My next infusion was moved to Friday. I am going to need the extra day to have the courage to go through this again.

Day 37: It Gets a Little Better

Last night was okay. I slept most of the night without pain. The drugs are working somewhat. I am okay lying or sitting down when my leg muscles aren't under tension. The problem with the leg muscles is when I am still for a period of time. Dakota got up around 2:30 am, a good time to take the meds and move my legs. I am feeling more like myself today.

Acupuncture and dinner out. Looking forward to both.

---

[3] Monkey bread is a sweet, sticky, pull-apart pastry made from small dough balls baked together in a bundt pan. Once baked, it's usually pulled apart piece by piece—exactly how I felt in that moment.

Day 38: Acupuncture and Chemo Acne

I am sitting on a bench outside, waiting in the glorious sun to go into the building for acupuncture. Acupuncture is still a bit of a mystery to me. It does help alleviate headaches, swelling, and other issues.

I sent some notes and asked more questions due to the state of my face. I continue to feel like a bit of a guinea pig as they try to deal with the side effects. The oncologist thinks the Gabapentin may have caused the acne[4]. So, we're stopping that drug. She is going to give me an oral steroid for a few days after chemo to see if that helps with the leg nerve issue. My blood counts were good today, so I am ready for the infusion tomorrow.

Then, week two of 12 will be done. After the 12 weeks, they will wait for three to four weeks with no infusions, and I will have a lumpectomy and reduction surgery. Depending on what they find during surgery, they will decide how much radiation I need and what ongoing infusions I may need.

---

[4] In retrospect, I don't think I took Gabapentin long enough or at a high enough dose to have it provide me with any relief. The steroids helped with the chemo acne and my energy level more than anything else they gave me.

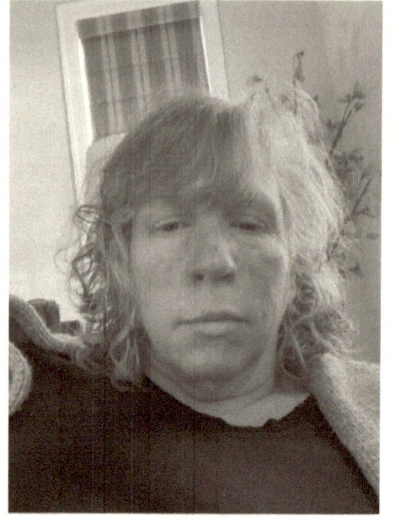

So, now I know that chemo acne or "chemo face" is a thing. I look like a teenager, all red and broken out across my cheeks and nose. And it hurts. The leg cramps have lessened, or maybe I am getting accustomed to the nerve pain. I see the oncologist at lunchtime today.

Gus dug out my shower chair (I used it after each of my four knee surgeries) so I can sit during my shower and while brushing my teeth. Standing still is still really uncomfortable.

I did not sleep at all last night. Dakota was breathing unevenly (he has congestive heart failure in addition to all his other issues), and I couldn't relax. I'm hoping to catch a nap before acupuncture later today.

The second Taxol infusion is tomorrow. Only one drug. Hoping it goes faster. The nurse said it would take an hour.

Day 39: Post-Chemo

Today was a pretty good day. I got up and finished packing my chemo bag. My face was still a mess, and I was happy to put on a mask. I put Lidocaine on my port and covered it with plastic wrap and tape to numb the skin.

It's funny; initially, I was so worried about how much it would hurt for them to access my port. But after the first few times, I realized it wasn't a big deal. Take a deep breath, and don't lean back to escape the needle. It's actually easier than a traditional IV.

I got all my stuff, and Gus drove me down. He had meetings, so I went in alone. I checked in and got the same nurse—Emma—from the week before. I found out I had two drugs today, and I got to be observed by four premedical students.

It took three hours. I was wrapped in my Talli Blanket, clutching my new Charlie the Chemo dog—a lavender-scented, weighted toy—and wearing my noise-canceling headphones.

I showed Emma my acne face, and she said she would ask around for ideas on what to do. I told her my prescription was not ready for tomorrow—a new drug to replace the first drug they had prescribed—and she said she'd take care of it. It can cause insomnia, so she wants me to take it as soon as I wake up. *Oh, the wonders of steroids!*

I was alert until the pre-medical Benadryl, and then I was dizzy and unable to stay awake.

Emma came back and gave me three things: 1) she called the pharmacy and asked them to release my prescription immediately—which they did, because I got a text right before I left; 2) she polled the Nurse Practitioners about my rash and told me to slather on hydrocortisone cream (over the counter); and 3) she told me to pick up some Press'n Seal-style plastic wrap—a cling film with a light adhesive backing—to help the lidocaine stay in place over my port.

I sent a note to my oncologist to see if they have a recognition program so I can get Emma some award for patient care. She is amazing. I also wanted my oncologist to add what I have learned from Emma and the other nurses to the binder they give to new patients. There is so much more they could tell you before you start treatment.

Update: My skin has almost cleared. I am thrilled. Steroids are scary, and a little magical.

I feel okay. I have an appetite. No nausea. I am moving around slowly. My body feels heavy and tired: nothing I cannot handle.

Day 40: The Miracle of Steroids

Last night was bad. I ended up lying in the recliner and did not sleep much. Today, I took the new med early and had a remarkably productive day. Steroids are miraculous. I got laundry done, the dishes done, my paper pile cleaned up, and I took a walk with Talli. I made dinner and cleaned up, and my legs aren't bothering me.

Rocking my short hair thanks to Sarah's skills, she learned from cutting her mom's hair during COVID. Grateful for friends who have stopped by, and for the food, which was helpful last week when we were overwhelmed. We had a wonderful dinner out with Kathy and Orlando. Kathy also spoiled us with some fantastic homemade pastries. No photo since they didn't last five minutes before we devoured them.

Enjoying the tulips and food Carrie and Dutch brought. The salad lasted me three meals, and the soup fed us for two.

I am doing okay today. My hair has not started to fall out yet, and my port is healing nicely without a big scar.

I walked nearly 23,000 steps today. Hoping for another good day tomorrow. The sun certainly helped today.

Day 45: Los Lobos

I went to see Los Lobos with Julia and Gus last night. The last time Gus and I saw them was when we lived in California. We think it was 32 years ago! Julia was the youngest person in Revolution Hall.

I had an enjoyable time and felt pretty good the whole time. I slept well last night, and my chemo bag is packed and ready. Julia is picking me up and dropping me off this morning for my infusion. Gus will pick me up later.

I am feeling good enough to do a VR workout. I want to exercise before my infusion so I can check it off my to-do list. I can't get through each day without having a list of things to do or accomplish. That includes some sort of exercise. VR is the most I can handle these days. My only complaint has been some tummy trouble the last few days. The headache dissipated earlier this week, so I was able to read a book and get some help on how to deal with my grief. It was a great book, with tactical advice that I have put into practice. My therapist is excellent. She helped a lot. This book was her recommendation. There isn't much new info for me. The helpful part is the way he helps you put the advice into practice daily.

Day 46: Chemo Three Done

The good news. Round three of chemo is done. This brings me to 25% complete.

Yesterday's infusion was a bit of a sh*t show. Julia dropped me off, and I got there on time.

They started with the blood draw, but my port wouldn't give them blood. It had clotted over. They had to put some stuff in my port to rotor-rooter (clean out) the line. So, they decided to try a traditional blood draw in my forearm to stay on schedule. They couldn't get a good draw since my veins roll, so I have another bruise and no blood to show for it. They abandoned trying to give me a traditional IV. Instead, they decided to wait for the port to clear. I was behind schedule. No chairs were available in the big room, so I ended up in one of the private rooms. As I have long suspected, having a private room is less efficient. It took a lot longer for them to get to me and push all the drugs. I only chased someone down once to ask about time, so I wasn't too obnoxious. I arrived at 9:30 am and left at 2:00 pm. They were clearly not adequately staffed for the number of patients requiring infusions today.

When Gus picked me up, I was just tired. Colleen had texted earlier with an acupuncture appointment, so Gus took me at 5:30 pm. That was helpful. I perked up and made dinner afterward. She also got my shoulder to stop bothering me—it was more of a muscular problem than anything else. Bonus!

I went to bed at 10 pm and took all the meds, even though I wasn't feeling bad. I thought I had gotten ahead of it.

The nausea isn't present now, and taking the meds earlier appears to have worked. I am up now at 3 am with diarrhea and cramps. I dug out my weighted blanket, took more meds, and hung out in Julia's bed, so I don't bug Gus and Dakota. The blanket's weight is comforting. I'm hoping I can fall back asleep—that my body can metabolize the meds and things quiet down.

Heartburn Storms

The meds took hold around 7 am, and I had a mostly bathroom-free day. Drank lots of electrolytes, cleaned the kitchen, and did the laundry. That feels like an accomplishment worth mentioning.

I played VR Mini Golf and some other games with Talli for a bit. Michelle sent some gorgeous flowers, which definitely lifted my spirits.

It snowed up here today. That was fun to watch. It's all melted now.

While I'm making dinner, I feel okay: just tired. My face is still flushed. I'm thinking I need to take the steroid tomorrow. I'll see if it keeps me from fully breaking out like a teenager.

I'm adding Prilosec to see if I can get ahead of the heartburn storm that's coming with next week's chemo. That will be all three drugs. This week was only one. Then, I'll be at 50% for the four major chemo weeks. Two down and two to go. I am running the numbers to help me get to the other side. It must be a project manager thing.

Gia offered to take care of dinner next week after the chemo. Thank you! One less thing for me to worry about.

Doing OK this evening. Hoping for a good night's sleep.

Day 47: More Acne

I'm feeling good today after having some insomnia last night. Got up early and took the steroid for my face. It got red again yesterday. It must be the Taxol. It didn't hurt or blister this time, so that was good. Got in a nice, long VR workout on the Oculus. Daisy and Gerber are here for a visit.[5]

---

[5] The two cute Chihuahuas in the photo on the next page belong to a friend of a friend. We love having them stay with us instead of being kenneled when their mom travels.

They'll stay until Tuesday. They make me laugh and smile. Unlike Dakota, they like the car. We went to Target to pick up my cleaning supply order. I think Gerber missed Gus. It's been a while since they spent time together. We love pet-sitting for Pam. Glad to be feeling good today.

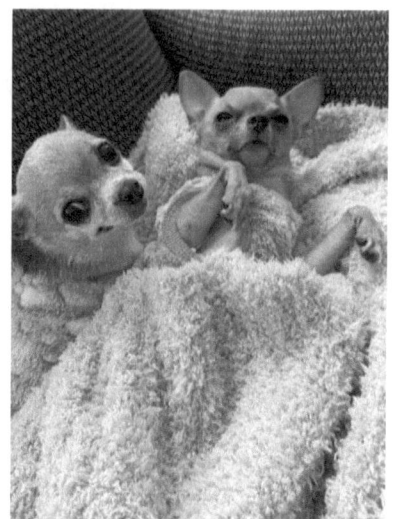

Day 49: Prepping for Second 3-Drug Chemo

One big chemo session down, and I was already learning how much preparation mattered. The second big round approached when I got all the drugs at once, and I was determined to do everything I could to make it more bearable.

I'm doing okay this morning, but I had a rough evening last night. My digestive tract is not happy with me.

Yesterday was good. I saw Vicki for lunch and enjoyed learning a new craft at Erin's. We decorated eggs with wax and dye. After some medication, I managed to sleep, even with Gerber wanting to get up on our bed in the middle of the night.

I worked out for 45 minutes in VR this morning. I love the Oculus and the Supernatural workout program. I have lost a few pounds over the last few weeks. I miss Pilates, but I am uncomfortable around sweaty, germy people. I can't afford to get sick.

I have a check-in with a friend from work today; I hope to get to Kornblatt's for a last lox bagel before they close. Tomorrow, I have a little work to do for an upcoming workshop I am giving in April. I also have my final therapy session with Dr. Michelle Lee, who has been really helpful.

All is going well into big chemo number two this week. I am nervous. But then I'll be 50% done with the big sessions and 33% done overall. I am getting acupuncture on Wednesday to see if that helps boost my blood count. I'm also adding more protein because Vicki says it helps with recovery, and I am working out every day to stay strong and focused.

Surviving Chemo

Infusion days have been long. I am hoping this week isn't too many hours. Noise-canceling headphones and snacks are getting me through. I have my lovely blanket from Talli and Charlie the Chemo dog. I have to sit with ice gloves and socks on during the Taxol part to see if we can stave off the neuropathy.

So far, the symptoms have been nerve pain in the back of my legs, diarrhea, nausea, exhaustion, and horrible facial acne that required steroids.

I am taking it slow since I don't know if my energy will continue to wax and wane or if I'll get increasingly tired as this goes along.

Off to lunch and hanging with the Chihuahuas.

Day 52: Chemo Acne

Tuesday night was awful. I was on the toilet every hour, on the hour. I ended up sleeping on the couch so Gus could get some sleep. Kept taking anti-diarrhea meds, but they didn't take hold until 5:30 am. I spent most of yesterday like a zombie, with that tired/exhausted/hungover/buzzy feeling all day. I have developed a rash over my back, and when I woke up this morning (after resorting to Xanax), my face had broken out again. I felt okay today, though. I worked out and cleaned the kitchen and bathroom. I went for chemo and had a lot of pre-game drugs for stomach, skin, and allergies. Then, all three chemo drugs and a hefty dose of Benadryl knocked out the rash. My face is getting better. I slept through most of the infusion. They woke me up for the drug changeover and line flushing. When I got home, I felt okay. I took some anti-nausea and anti-diarrhea meds early and then again before bed. I made dinner, and now I feel OK. Mild headache this time.

My hair started falling out in the shower this morning. I hope it stays long enough for me to conduct a paid workshop on Tuesday. Then, I will ask Sarah to cut it even shorter, as I prepare to shave it off.

Tomorrow, I am going to try to groom Dakota. He's had such bad luck with groomers. The last one nicked his eye and gave him an ulcer that had to be treated with drops that affected his heart. I will go slow and, even if it takes all day, get him down to less hair. I want to see if it helps his skin heal. His allergies are flaring, and he's biting himself to the point of infection. Nothing is working.

I'll be on Amazon next. I hear I need to order a bed wedge to help me sleep.

Day 56: Hair Fall

My hair falling out in the shower was shocking this morning. I will be bald by the weekend, if not before. I am out today wearing a hat. It's crazy how dead my hair feels.

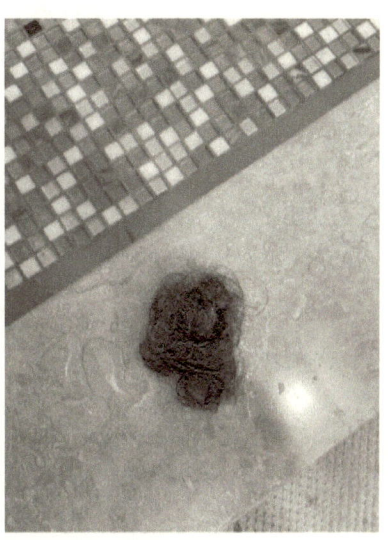

I am delivering the workshop tomorrow afternoon. The big debate is whether to wear a hat or try out the wig with what's left of my hair. Neither option feels good.

Day 57: Shaved My Head

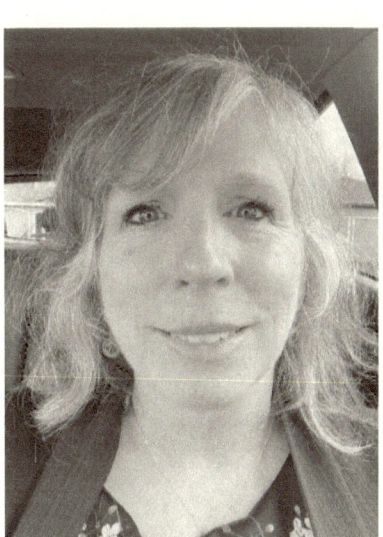

Today was hard and good at the same time. I spent the morning printing and preparing for the workshop I gave this afternoon. Washing my hair has become an ordeal. Clumps are falling out, tangling in my fingers and my rings. It looks like a small animal died in the shower. I didn't realize how many strands are on my head until I started losing them. Gus assured me I didn't look bad, and I went without a hat or wig, sporting my shoulder-length hair that Sarah cleaned up after I cut a foot or more of hair off myself in the bathroom.

It was nerve-wracking as I stood before 40 women and gave my presentation. I had a hard time focusing because I thought I could feel my hair falling out while I was leading the workshop. I used a ton of hairspray. Afterward, people came up to chat, picking stray hairs off my dress and shoulders, as women do. "Oh, you're shedding. Let me get that for you," someone said.

Nonetheless, the workshop went really well. I got some great comments, and I think I've got some work to do. I saw some old colleagues and new friends from the last event I attended. It was lovely, at least when I managed to get out of my head and stop obsessing about the hair.

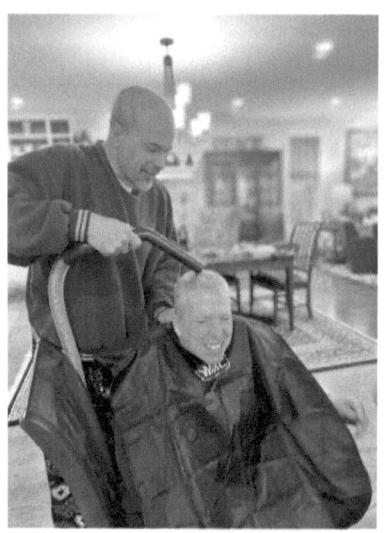

As soon as I left the event, I called Talli and Sarah and asked them to come to the house for pizza and a buzz cut. With pizza on the counter, I sat on a chair dragged into the kitchen to avoid any mirrors. Gus was armed with the vacuum, Sarah shaved my head, while Talli took videos and pictures. I didn't want to watch. I laughed and held it together as the last of my hair fell to the floor, and Gus efficiently sucked it all into the vacuum before I could see.

I'm grateful to all three of them for supporting me through the transition to near baldness.

Tomorrow's shower should not be traumatic. I need to remember I don't need a lot of shampoo.

It's cold and drafty without the hair. What a shock to the system. I am so glad to have a partner and friends who have distracted me and made me laugh.

I will show off some of the wigs in the coming days. And now I need to get my eyebrows micro bladed. I am feeling pretty naked. Oh, and perhaps false eyelashes. I'll need Claire's help working them out.

Day 58: Five of Twelve

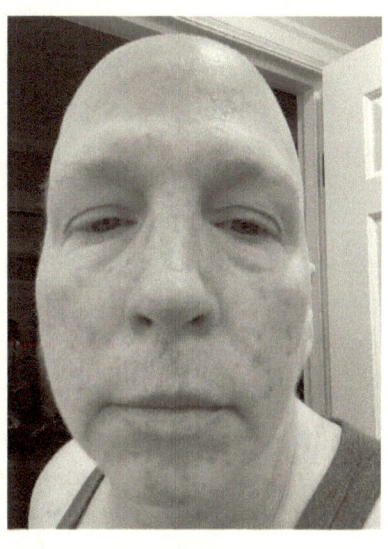

Chemo Infusion 5 of 12 is done! Ursula took me down to my appointment. Everything was smooth. It took four hours. The oncologist came to see me and reduced the dosage because I am experiencing neuropathy in the tips of my fingers. She doesn't want it to become permanent. I wore my frozen mittens to see if we can stop the nerves from being destroyed. She also hopes the reduction will reduce my need for steroids to combat the chemo acne.

Gus picked me up around two pm; I watched far too much TV and was so tired I barely moved. Molly brought dinner and breakfast for tomorrow. The enchiladas were fantastic.

Then Carrie brought her new puppy, Lola. She's so much smaller than I expected for a Bernedoodle. And so cute! She perked me up, and I felt okay as I got ready for bed. Dakota wasn't a fan. He is overwhelmed by puppy energy.

I'm going to eat some Tums and see if that keeps the heartburn at bay. Following mom's advice and taking only the peppermint-flavored ones. They seem to be more effective than the other flavors.

I haven't tried to lie horizontally yet. That's usually when the trouble starts. I have the new bolster (wedge) from Amazon to put under my upper body. I'm going to try that tonight.

Next week, I will be halfway done with chemo. And the week after is my mid-point ultrasound to see if the tumor has shrunk.

I'm grateful to see friends and talk about normal stuff.

Day 62: A Moment of Normalcy

Happy Easter. Ours was very low-key. Claire worked late last night and had to be back at work for a shift today, so we missed seeing her. Julia, Gus, and I went to the Cadillac Cafe in Northeast Portland for breakfast. It was nice. First time out with a wig. What's left of my hair continues to wither and die on my head. It's like straw, dropping off everywhere.

I feel much better after last week's lower dose of Taxol. The 20% reduction significantly affected the amount of energy I had and how my system responded to the infusion. I am sleeping better, too. We're still sticking close to home most of the time, to keep germs to a minimum. I have been doing pick-ups at Target and the pharmacy drive-thru to minimize my time around strangers. I continue to do my workouts with the Oculus. I sweat and get good cardio every day.

Limbo land. That's where I feel I am. Trying to keep my blood cell count high enough to take the treatment, to stay as healthy and strong as I can, while I continue down this crazy countdown until the end of chemo.

This is a milestone week—my sixth treatment, and I'll be 50% done by Thursday afternoon. Then the next big thing is a week later, on April 19—I'll be getting a follow-up ultrasound to measure the tumor and see if it's shrinking. I'll know immediately if the chemo shrank the tumor, since my doctor's appointment is right after the ultrasound.

Grateful for **Ursula**, who is my ride down to the hospital each week. That's taken a huge burden off of Gus.

Grateful for **Michelle**, who called today and dealt with my phone battery dying and then the house phone going out, so we could have a long catch-up on life. It's so good to have an everyday conversation about normal things. I am hoping we can drive down to southern Oregon to see her new house and meet the new dog, Dharma.

I hope everyone had a lovely Passover and Easter and is enjoying seeing the flowers bloom. Spring shows her lovely face, even if it's been extremely wet in Oregon. At least the drought may be a thing of the past, since we've had so much rain and snow.

I am hopeful the treatment is working and that in seven more weeks, my hair will begin to grow, and I'll be preparing for surgery and life on the other side of this ordeal.

Day 70: New Socks, No Hair

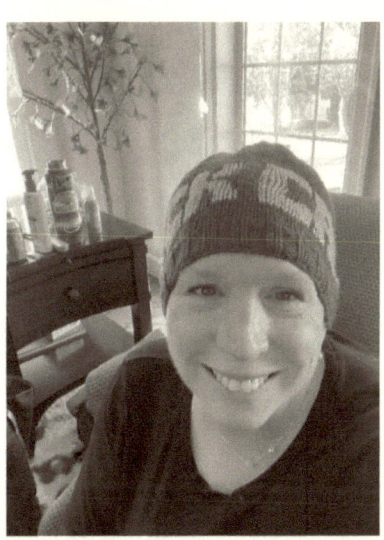

This has been a rough week. The exhaustion is non-stop. I can barely keep my head up most of the day. I managed to get out to dinner with Vicki yesterday and had an exploratory meeting for some consulting today. Then I came home and collapsed on the couch. I feel like I am running at 20%. I got some great new chemo socks from Talli. I can't wait to wear them on Thursday. I also wore my knit cap (F*ck Cancer), which I got from Michelle last week. She used the same yarn she uses for all the new babies in her family. The nurses loved it. And it kept my head warm.

This week, we will shave off the little hair I have left, and I will get a henna crown on my bald dome on Friday. That should be fun.

I am so tired of being tired. I can't hold my head up this evening. I am barely doing the minimum to keep Dakota from making a mess in the house. Please send me some strength. I am not feeling up to the task of being a good patient today. This cumulative response is getting to me. I was hoping it would be more of a rollercoaster. Instead, I keep feeling worse. Praying for an up day tomorrow.

Day 72: MRI Update – Tumor Shrunk!

> *When I thought ahead to hearing those words— "the tumor has shrunk"—I expected relief. Instead, I felt a mix of exhaustion, disbelief, and a cautious hope that I barely allowed myself to feel. Cancer really teaches you not to celebrate too soon.*

Good news today. The tumor has shrunk.[6] The tech struggled to find it. The next step is to complete chemo. Six more weekly treatments. Then, a few weeks to let the body recover. Then, surgery in mid-late June. Then, sixteen daily radiation treatments. I am not sure I have processed what it all means.

Thanks for the tumor-shrinking dances. They worked!

Tomorrow is the third of the four big chemos. All three drugs. Sigh. One day at a time.

As treatment continued, the rhythms of chemo started to feel both familiar and unbearable. Each week had its own routine, its own dread, its own countdown. I kept to myself in the infusion room, trying to get through the hours without thinking too far ahead. But in the middle of all that isolation, something unexpected happened. One ordinary treatment day, a woman walked in and changed the way I saw the entire journey.

---

[6] FINDINGS: The known invasive carcinoma corresponds to an irregular hypoechoic 0.8 x 0.7 x 0.6 cm mass with an associated localizer device at 2:00, 13 cm from the nipple, previously 1.1 x 1.2 x 1.6 cm. No new masses are seen in the region.

The Unexpected Mentor

One of those long chemo days arrived, and as soon as I walked into the infusion room, I sensed that something about the space felt different. Two chairs were directly in front of me, with the curtains pulled on both sides, creating a small pod. Most days, the curtains were open, giving the nurses a clearer view of our machines and our faces. It also made it easier for them to check on us quickly. Having the curtains pulled felt unusual, more private, almost as if the room were giving us permission to hide.

I sat down in one of the chairs, bald, masked, exhausted, and doing my best to brace myself for another long session. A few minutes later, a woman who looked a few years older than me walked in with a spring in her step. She had the sharpest short salt-and-pepper haircut I had ever seen. She looked chic and light, as if she had somehow escaped the heaviness that had taken over my body. She slipped into the chair next to mine, both of us still able to see out into the room even with the curtains creating our little enclosure.

I had barely spoken to anyone in the infusion room up to this point. I kept my head down and tried to survive each week. But something about her made me reach for courage. So I asked, "May I ask you a question?"

She smiled and said yes.

"Are you here for breast cancer treatment?"

"Oh, I'm here for an infusion after breast cancer," she said. "Kadcyla today."

I didn't know it then, but that was something I would also need later. I asked where she was in her journey, and she told me she had finished chemotherapy, completed surgery, completed radiation, and had just come from a follow-up with her plastic surgeon.

I asked the question I was scared to ask out loud. "Can you give me a sense of how long it took to grow your hair out that far?" Hair had always mattered to me. Losing it stripped something away I wasn't prepared for. And here she was, sitting casually beside me, looking like the woman I used to be and desperately wanted to become again.

She told me she was about five months out from her first chemotherapy treatment. That small piece of information did more for me than any pamphlet or doctor's explanation ever had.

Then she asked who my surgeon was. I said Nathalie Johnson. She said, "She's my surgeon." Then she asked about my plastic surgeon. I said Kyle Baltrusch. "He's mine too," she laughed. "In fact, I was with him today. He told me my breasts were so spectacular that he wants to put my before-and-after photos on the website. You want to see them?"

Before I could respond, she pulled the curtain in front of us closed, lifted her top, and flashed me. No bra. Full reveal. I burst out laughing. It was the first time in weeks I felt anything close to joy. I told her they looked spectacular. She grinned, said, "Right?" and dropped the curtain back open like nothing unusual had happened.

A nurse walked over to hook up her adjunct therapy while another nurse let me know my blood work had come back, and they were preparing my chemo. It struck me how two people could be in the exact same room, in the exact same

38

chairs, but be living completely different chapters of the same story. She was ahead of me. She had made it through. And seeing her—really seeing her—made me believe I could get there too.

What I want readers to take away from this moment is simple: we need mentors. We need them at work, and we need them through illness. They show up as therapists, doctors, other patients, loved ones, and even strangers who sit next to us in infusion pods with short, perfect hair and zero hesitation about flashing their reconstructed breasts.

I realized I had been isolating myself because I didn't want to bother anyone. But by keeping quiet, I was cutting myself off from the exact people who could help me learn, hope, and prepare for what was coming. That woman gave me perspective and strength when I had none left. She gave me something to look toward.

There were others, too. Erin H. answered my questions, gave me things I didn't know I needed, and told me I could get through it. Amber reminded me to go one step at a time and soon I would be on the other side. My therapist helped me remember to be kind to myself. My doctors reminded me they were continuously researching and putting me on the best path forward.

When you are in the middle of treatment, you cannot see the end. You cannot see the light at the end of the tunnel, or the finish line, or the version of yourself who is recovering, healing, and growing hair again. It feels endless. But others have walked this path. They know the turns. They know the dark spots. They can tell you where the ground is when you can't feel it.

If you are a patient, think about who you can reach out to. Also, think about who might need your experience. And if you are supporting someone through cancer, consider how you might help them find mentors who can hold what you can't. You are not expected to know everything. You are not expected to carry it alone.

There is a whole community of women who have been through this, and they are generous with their stories because they know how much those stories matter. Let them help you find hope again.

Reflection Prompt:

Who has walked this path before you? Who can you learn from? And who, even in your hardest moments, might need your voice and your courage to guide them forward?

Chapter 3: Medical Crisis

Just when I thought I couldn't feel more tired, I did. And I thought that by putting one foot in front of the other, I would get to the end without anything new adding to my stress and discomfort. I was about to learn how important it is to listen to my body and interpret what my watch was trying to tell me.

Day 73: Skipping Chemo – Going Downhill

Damn it. I am too sick and run down to take chemo this week. This means I will have to tack on another week. The oncologist ran a bunch of extra bloodwork, and I am sitting here getting a bag of fluids. Ugh. So disappointed. I didn't want to extend a week. Intellectually, I understand their reasons. I have been half-dead this last week.

I need to keep up the protein and fluids so I can get back on track next week. Maybe this horrible rash and itchiness on my back and upper thighs will also have a chance to clear.

After I got home, I went on Reddit and described my symptoms since I am feeling worse. They've all advised me to call my doctor immediately and consider a trip to the ER.

F*ck cancer.

Day 74: Hospitalization for Blood Clot

Hello from the ER. It turns out I have a clot (pulmonary embolism or PE for short) in my lung. Those women on Reddit were right. It was more serious than I believed.

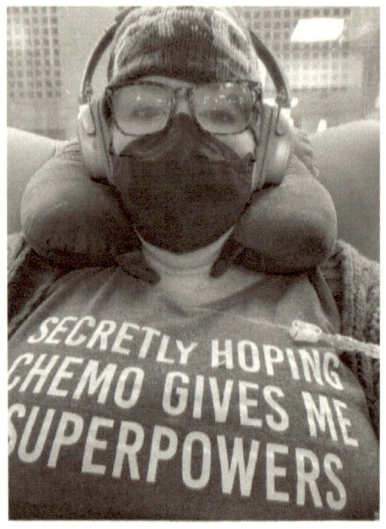

Waiting to see if they will keep me overnight. Explains the shortness of breath and feeling like garbage.

They are running additional tests.

I have a fever. I can't seem to cool off. The nurse hung fluids. Just waiting. Hopefully, I will get to go home. I had to cancel my appointment for my henna crown.

Update: I'm spending the night at St Vincent's Hospital. Room 18, after a shot in the stomach with a blood thinner. They have me hooked up to a heart monitor. The fever is down, but not gone. They pulled more blood for a culture. We will find out more tomorrow. I'm going to try to sleep. Gus is home with Dakota. Julia packed me a bag of stuff to get me through. I got my Talli Blanket and Charlie, the Chemo dog. Thanks for coming, Talli and Erin. Gus – you're a rock star. Sorry to mess up your birthday. We will reschedule. I love you. Xoxo

Day 76: Home Again

I am home. I went in on Friday with shortness of breath and found out I had a blood clot in my right lung. Now, I need to take blood thinners for the next three months.[7]

---

[7] Note: I am still on blood thinners nearly two years later. Tamoxifen can cause blood clots, so they kept me on it due to an abundance of caution. Tamoxifen (a brand name for tamoxifen citrate) is commonly used in hormone therapy for 5-10 years after

They ruled out a bunch of stuff, with urine, blood, and stool samples and cultures. They can't figure out why I had a fever of 99-102.

I believe they checked me out thoroughly. It is so good to be home.

Update: This is a longer post to explain the events of the past few days in more detail. I couldn't have dreamt it up.

Friday (Day 74) started with Gus and me taking Dakota to the vet. Dakota has a heart murmur, and his heart is failing slowly. He takes medication for his heart to help it pump more efficiently. He is also having trouble with his kidneys. So, he takes Lasix to make him pee more. The vet is trying to balance out his meds to support his heart and kidneys. So, blood tests are how we keep an eye on what's going on with him. Friday was a regular blood test. Dakota is having trouble eating, too. So, we're handfeeding him. He's going blind, is mostly deaf, and still has a good appetite. He has difficulty finding his plate and eating efficiently without help.

So, on Friday, we are on the way to the vet when I realize I am having trouble breathing. I asked some questions on Reddit. They advised going to the ER. So, after talking to the oncology team, that's the plan – get Dakota tested, bring him home, and then go to St. Vincent's (close to the house). Gus went in with him and waited in the waiting room, where he could hear Dakota yelling. His veins were difficult to access because he hadn't had much for breakfast, and he was dehydrated.

After we got out of there, I started to drive us all home. As we got closer to home, Dakota got antsy; it was as if he had

---

active treatment to keep the estrogen and progesterone low in my body to starve any cancer that may reappear. Remember, I had triple-positive breast cancer. It feeds off of estrogen and progesterone.

to go to the bathroom. As we didn't want him to poop in the car, I pulled over at Mill Pond Park and crossed the street with him because he likes grass. I kept blocking him to keep him in the right spot. He got irritated with me and stepped back fast over the edge of the hill.

I watched him tumble down the very steep embankment. It's grass and mud, so he'd stop for a second and then tumble some more. I yelled at Gus, who got out of the car and went after him. Gus managed to stay on his feet about 50% of the way down, and then he fell on his butt and slid the rest of the way. He captured Dakota, and we headed home.

Dakota didn't seem worse for wear – just muddy and with burrs in his fur. My breathing continued to worsen, so we quickly dropped Dakota off, then Gus changed his clothes, and we headed to the ER.

St Vincent's wasn't terribly busy, but there were more people than I was comfortable sitting with without a mask. I ended up asking two people to put their masks on as I explained that I have cancer and am immunocompromised. Both were apologetic and complied or left the area.

After triage, we waited about 45 minutes and were taken back to a room. The doctor was in quickly and asked me a bunch of questions. When I suggested I had pneumonia (as it felt similar to my bout of pneumonia, most likely from SARS, 20 years ago), he said, "No, it is more likely that you have a blood clot in your lungs." He ordered a CT scan, and his suspicion was quickly validated.

He told me I needed to be admitted for observation. We waited until about seven pm, and then I got a room. They accessed my port and pulled blood for tests. At around one pm, Gus got a frantic call from our house cleaner. Dakota had his neck wrapped in Gus's wired headset (no wireless headset can last a full day for Gus). He had then freaked out and pooped under Gus's desk while he was stuck and appeared to be hanging himself slowly. She couldn't get close to him, as he grew more frantic as she approached, and she didn't want the cord to get any tighter. Gus raced home (sorry, neighbors), disentangled Dakota, and then locked him out of the office after cleaning up the poop. (I was thinking, "Like, is this real? How much more sh*t can we deal with this week?")

I spent two nights in the hospital, with wonderful nurses. They poked me, took my blood pressure, and checked my temperature and my oxygen levels every hour the first night. Last night, they let me sleep. They were worried because my fever kept spiking. I was okay, then it was 99. Then it was 101, then it was normal. And then back up again. So, they took more things to test. Blood from my arm (in case my port was compromised. So, I got two nice bruises on my left arm because not all nurses are trained to use a medical infusion port.) Urine. Stool. Everything came back okay this morning, and the cultures hadn't grown anything yet (taken on Friday), so the doctor said I could go home. However, I am no longer allowed to take anything that contains aspirin.

I need to walk every day. I am going to tag along with the Herreras and their dog Koda on their regular lunch walk to see if that keeps me moving. I will be on blood thinners (oral, thank goodness) for the next three months. They started me on belly shots/injections, and that was freaking miserable. Belly shots hurt when they go in and burn as they move around your stomach fat. I am so glad he moved me to a pill.

I am doing okay and so relieved to be home. I need to make Dakota's food today. I have him on a fish diet with a lot of veggies and supplements. It still feels weird to take deep breaths. I understand the clot could take weeks to dissolve. The drugs are to make sure it doesn't grow and that others don't form.

As I left, they flushed my port with Heparin. I need to be double-sure not to hit myself on anything or fall down (I am a klutz). So, I am moving slowly and carefully to avoid bruising.

The last few days really drove home how much I dislike being out of my house and away from Gus and Dakota. What a lonely place the hospital is. Thank you to everyone who visited: Talli, Erin, Carrie! It meant a lot and helped when Gus couldn't be there.

Thanks for reading. It helps me when I can put all of this out there in writing. Have a wonderful Sunday!

I also dig into advocating for yourself in Chapter 21, and my friend Gail shares her own experience with it in Chapter 16.

Day 78: Dog Walking

Today, I am feeling better. It still hurts to fully inflate my lungs. Yesterday, I walked with Kathy and Koda. Today, Orlando joined us. On yesterday's walk, I was struggling a lot: I kept stopping and gasping for air. I had to put my head between my knees so I wouldn't pass out. Today was much better. I was still gasping and needed to slow down. But I had a much easier time walking. I'm going to keep at it every day and see if it continues to help my lungs inflate and reduce the clot's size.

I took my last dose of Tylenol yesterday. I am waiting to see if the fever returns. So far, I am getting a normal reading. The mysterious fever is still a mystery. I met my primary care doctor via video yesterday, and she said the cultures are still not showing any growth. So those should come back clean, too. If I continue to improve, I can have the chemo on Thursday.

I went to the chiropractor to get adjusted. My neck and hip were bugging me after sleeping in the hospital bed. I also got a massage. I am feeling so much better this evening.

Dakota gave us quite a scare today. He started to tremble and got strongly agitated. I gave him some doggie CBD, and Julia came up to hang out with him while I got my massage. He's only eating if we mix his food with baby food. Beef with gravy seems to do the trick. He's better this evening, and we're snuggled on the couch.

Day 80: After the Blood Clot

The rollercoaster ride continues. I have managed to walk every day this week. My blood oxygen is slowly coming up. I reached 99% O_2 saturation this morning. That's a first since this crazy ride started. My Apple Watch alerted me to an issue with my resting heart rate (RHR) last Tuesday. I received 58 reminders from Tuesday to Friday, stating that I was inactive and my RHR exceeded 100. That was the sign that I was struggling to get enough oxygen into my lungs, a strong indication I had a pulmonary embolism (PE) or blood clot. I wish I had paid attention sooner to what it was trying to tell me.

Yesterday, I felt pretty good until the afternoon when the headache roared back. I still don't know what the trigger is.

I took a few Tylenols and put some ice on my head, and it finally cleared up before bed. My mystery fever is still gone. I haven't had a fever all week. The last of the blood cultures showed up in MyChart: no sign of infection. Nothing grew in either sample.

I had an excellent lunch and walk with Lynn yesterday. Turns out Gus likes arugula salad.

Vicki came by with a favorite Iranian dinner: chicken eggplant with crunchy rice. And another salad Gus loved.

I am about to finish packing for chemo: the third long one today. All three drugs. Ursula is dropping me off. My headphones are charged. I am ready to zone out.

Enjoy the sun! Koda and I walked with Orlando this morning, and the weather was perfect! And the flowering trees, bushes, and bulbs are stunning.

Chapter 4: Life Goes On, Even During Treatment

Saying goodbye to Dakota in the middle of my cancer battle felt unbearably cruel. He had been my constant shadow, my silent comfort, and the one who stayed by my side through all of it. Letting go of him while fighting to hold onto my own life felt impossible.

Day 81: 75% Complete

I'm feeling good this morning, after a decent sleep. I pre-gamed with a lot of anti-nausea and diarrhea meds yesterday. So far, my GI tract is behaving.

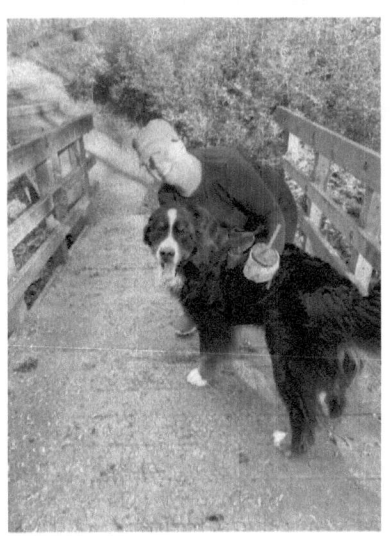

I'm dressed and ready for my walk with Koda (Orlando and Kathy's giant Burnese Mountain Dog). I love it that he moves at my current pace.

My lungs still feel like they are improving. It's a gorgeous day in Portland. I am going to put my hammock frame together so I can sit under the trees.

Stats: 75% complete with the three-drug chemo. Seven of the 12 chemo sessions are finished. Surgery is scheduled for June 30. I am on the downslope! F*ck cancer!

Day 88: Saying Goodbye

Checking in. Yesterday was chemo number eight out of 12. I am now 75% done. Everything went okay, but I am feeling exhausted, as expected. Otherwise, it's pretty routine. I was in and out reasonably quickly. Four more to go. I'll be done on June 1. Then I will heal for a month and have surgery on June 30.

June will mostly be free of appointments. I would love to get some lunches and dinners with friends on the books. Schedule me now.

We took Dakota to the vet for his weekly blood test. We've been watching him closely because of his kidneys and heart. He's been suffering from both congestive heart failure and kidney failure for a while. We've managed to keep him balanced on the stats with homemade food and medication. We found out this week that his kidneys are failing. We are going to put him to sleep here at home tomorrow. They are worried he's going to be in pain soon based on his blood work. His dementia continues to get worse. He's mostly blind and deaf as well. I am heartbroken and can't imagine getting through the rest of the year without him.

His little body can't take much more, and it's time. The girls are coming up to be with us as we say goodbye.

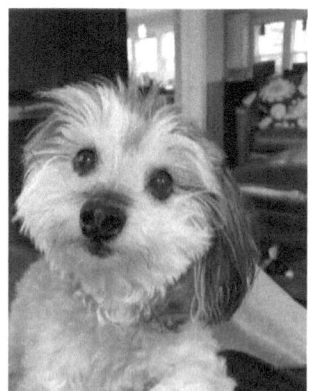

When Claire was a baby, we let our cat go too long with bad kidneys, and the end was awful for him. We can't let Dakota go through that experience or pain.

Hold Dakota and us in your hearts this weekend.

Day 98: Kiwi Head

It's Monday. Last week went okay as far as chemo is concerned. Struggling with energy levels, and yesterday, I was grateful we decided to stay home for Mother's Day brunch. The girls came over, cooked, and hung out; we had a lovely time. Being close to a bathroom is critical these days.

Sundays seem to be particularly bad for my gut health. I am plotting how to get my GI track back to normal after I am done on June 1. There are a lot of things they don't want me to mix with the chemo (including prebiotics and omega-3s), so I am waiting to take my regular supplements until after the chemo drugs have left my system. Imodium has become a new food group for me these past few weeks.

Lots of soup, flowers, orchids, a necklace, a journal, an impromptu dinner, and a beautiful watercolor of Dakota were delivered over these past few weeks. We are incredibly grateful to all of you who have been supporting us through chemo. Ursula is still driving me down each week. It's hard to believe there are only three more sessions to go.

This week will be a big one—three drugs, and then the last two weeks are chemo only. My head is fuzzy with hair. Gus thinks my head looks and feels like a kiwi fruit. I still have eyebrows (sparse) and eyelashes, and the hair on my head continues to grow, despite all the drugs. I have been rubbing rosemary oil into my scalp each night. It feels good on my dry skin, and it's supposed to help with growth. Notably, the white hairs are growing faster than the darker ones. I am concerned I'll be more grey than I was before this all started. It'll also be interesting to see if my hair grows faster after we stop the chemo drugs.

Tomorrow, I am sitting on a panel and will be out in public wearing a wig. It will feel weird, since I've been hiding for so many weeks. Looking forward to June, as I recover from the chemo and get ready for surgery on June 30. I get four weeks of no infusions. That's going to be different. I'll be meeting with my breast surgeon and the plastic surgeon. I am not sure when I will meet the radiation doctor. I am sure that's coming since I need to do 16 sessions after surgery. From what I understand, they'll be 10 minutes each, every weekday, for just over 3 weeks. It'll be in the basement of the same building where I have been going for chemo.

My breathing continues to be labored right after chemo, with a high resting heart rate, and then, as I get to Monday, it starts to come down. I appreciate my Apple Watch and all the data it provides. I feel less crazy now that I can see what's happening and watch the trends. I am praying there is no permanent damage to my organs from all the stuff 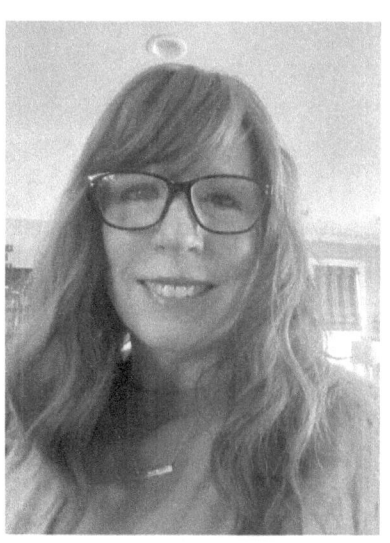 they've been drip-feeding into me these past nine weeks.

I wish you a lovely week and hope to see you soon!

Day 102: Postmenopausal

I can't sleep. I've been up since three am. Yesterday, I completed my final triple-drug chemo treatment. #10 out of 12 weeks done. Two more to go. Before I had my infusion, we met with the oncologist. It was a very emotional visit for me. She ordered a blood test to confirm my postmenopausal status. I just saw the test results come through in MyChart, confirming what I suspected – I am fully postmenopausal. That's good news for ongoing treatment. There are fewer hormones in my body to feed my triple-positive cancer.

What freaked me out yesterday was finding out that I need to take oral drugs for the next five to 10 years.[8] Cancer will be a part of my life, even though I will have completed chemo, surgery, and radiation in 2023.

Everything is pointing to the cancer having been killed off by the chemo. I will be cured. However, to ensure it doesn't come back or settle in a different part of my body, I must take *Tamoxifen* or a similar drug daily. I must also complete a full year of immunotherapy infusions every three weeks. So even though chemo is ending, I am not even close to being done.

I am back in active grief, with anger, denial, bargaining, and depression. This really sucks.

And to top it all off, I think I have a UTI. I was treated for a yeast infection last week. I don't think that was the problem now. I made an appointment for ZoomCare this morning to see if we can figure this out. It also could be strep from when I was in the hospital. The itchy and burning sensation keeps me from settling, so I can't sleep or relax.

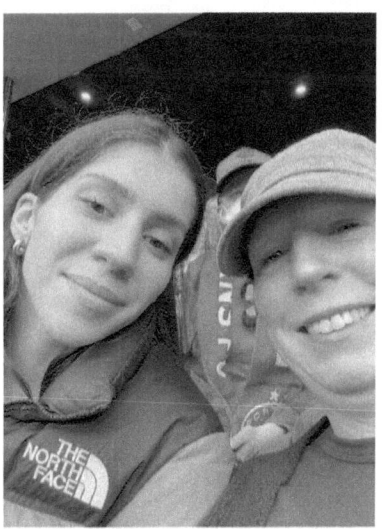

Julia and I are going to see Matchbox 20 tonight. I sure hope I can enjoy it.

In a few days, Claire and I are going to see a soccer

---

[8] This is when I learned that I would need to take a pill – Tamoxifen every day for the next ten years. I now see the drug as a medication that keeps me healthy. My sister helped me shift my thinking, and I am grateful to her for the coaching.

match at Providence Park. I sure miss playing. I am looking forward to spending some time with her.

Day 115: The Last Chemo

Today is my last chemo infusion. #12 of 12. It is hard to believe it's finally here. The last two weeks have been rough on my body and spirit. I haven't ventured far from the house, especially on Sundays and Mondays. I have had a few near misses because I wasn't close enough to a bathroom. My brain also feels scrambled. My taste buds are messed up, and my eyelashes are almost gone. The hair on my head is stubbornly growing back, so I have multi-colored stubble.

I have managed to get out a few times. We went and saw a house in Vancouver. It wasn't for us. We'll keep looking with Carrie W's help. We want to downsize and move to Washington State (less taxes!). I made it out to a few concerts. Last night was The Cure. Great show – and I'm so glad we were seated for most of it. I watched the folks who paid for floor seats—they had to stand for the entire three hours!

Today, I finished taking Taxol. I'll continue to take the other two drugs (Perjeta and Herceptin) every three weeks until I complete a year of treatment next winter. They've already put two sessions on my calendar. I hope that the sessions are easier on my body without the Taxol. The first immunotherapy-only infusion is on June 8.[9]

I'll spend this week (and probably next) recovering from this last dose of chemo. Then, I have the month to get stronger and ready for surgery. I have a few appointments before then. Meetings with the surgeons and a post-chemo echo of my heart, to compare it to the pre-chemo echo. I also

[9] Note: due to my advanced osteoporosis and the blood clots, I was actually put on Kadcyla instead of Perjeta and Herceptin.

have some lunches and meetings with friends to look forward to.

I expand on practical ways to support someone going through treatment in Chapter 28.

On June 10, we pick up our first foster dog. She's older and already house-trained. She was abandoned for a year before someone took her to the shelter. She's small, and we'll have fun guessing what she is. They think she's a Chihuahua mixed with a dachshund. They think she's around nine. Then, in July, our two little Chihuahua friends will be coming for a four-day visit while their mom is out of town. It's fun being the 'kennel' she drops them off at. We're both looking forward to having dog energy in the house again.

After surgery, I'll have radiation. We won't know how many sessions until the pathology comes back on my tumor after the surgery. So, that means more waiting. That'll also let us know what type of drug I need to be on for the next five to 10 years.

The infusion starts later today at 12:45 pm. I should be home by 4 pm.

Chapter 5: Surgery and Radiation

The night before surgery, I couldn't write a Facebook post. All I could do was try to mentally prepare. I lay awake, trying to convince myself that, in a few hours, this tumor would be gone. Surgery would mark another milestone, a victory. And yet, the fear remained—of complications, of the unknown, and of what my body would feel like when I woke up. I tried to accept the thought that this was a step toward healing. But sleep didn't come easily.

Day 135: Preparing for Surgery

Next Friday is my surgery date. I have to be at the hospital at 5:30 am for the lumpectomy, followed by a bilateral breast reduction. I'm excited to lose a few pounds, alleviate the strain on my back and neck, and get rid of whatever is left of the tumor. Hoping it's not much since it responded so well to treatment. Also, they will pull a few lymph nodes to ensure the cancer didn't spread from my breast.

See Section Six for checklists of what to bring and how to prepare.

Last week, I met with both the surgeon and the plastic surgeon, and I am confident they'll do a great job.

Gus is back in Florida. His mom is not well. He's her advocate and needs to be down there. I am alone with Tapi, the foster dog.[10] She is lovely, quiet, and a good companion. I would love to see any of you for lunch, dinner, or tea. Let me know if you have time.

I will pick Gus up at the airport next Wednesday. I don't have much on my calendar.

I had a lovely lunch with Cyrene yesterday and have a happy hour planned with Carrie on Thursday. I saw Stephanie last week and am still enjoying the flowers she brought. The biscotti are long gone, but they inspired me to bake some of my own. I hope to see Sarah this weekend. And Julia stopped by today with a chai.

My brain fog appears to be lifting. My taste buds are still messed up. My sister, Ali, advises giving them at least four months to recover. I have a halo of white hair growing in. My eyebrows are still sparse. My eyelashes are also thin. However, I have all sorts of serums and potions to help them grow.

I have more energy. I'm not at 100%, but I'm feeling better. My intestinal issues continue. I am trying to get it under control with probiotics and more fiber-rich foods.

I took on a house project last week. We got the roof replaced, gutters up and down, new soffits up for more airflow, and a fence between the neighbors and me repaired. I scheduled the paint touch-up, and we also need to power-wash the pergola. So, the house looks good.

Wishing you all a lovely summer solstice. I can't believe it's here already: the longest day of the year. Sunset is at 9:05 pm. Happy Half-Birthday, Julia!

---

[10] While no dog could ever take Dakota's place, I needed to have dog energy in the house. Gus and I discussed it for a while and decided to foster instead of adopting right away. Tapi was one of two fosters we helped find new homes for until Georgie came along and we adopted her on the spot.

Day 145: The Day after Surgery

Good morning! Yesterday, I was too out of it to write. I couldn't keep my eyes open after surgery. Julia came on Thursday night to sleep in her old room with Tapi. Tapi moaned until Julia took her back to our room at 4:45 am. Tapi has someone interested in adopting her. We will see if they can meet up this weekend. Time for this sweet pup to get a permanent home. She's very hairy. Dropping it everywhere. We are not used to it, as Dakota didn't shed at all. It's so strange to see it all over my pants and the couch. That makes me think I should be vacuuming more often. I don't have the energy for it.

We got to the hospital early. They checked me in and put Gus's phone number in the system so they could reach him later.

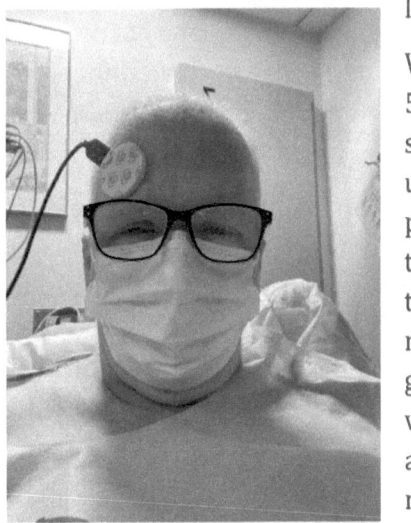

We waited a while past the 5:30 a.m. check-in time for someone to come and get us. We went back to the prep area and did all the things. The body temperature probe is on my head. Funny paper gown that heats you up with air. My anti-slip socks are red. The color lets the nurses know I don't walk well when medicated due to my previous leg injury. For the IV, she got it on the first try, using one of those machines where you can see the veins with light. Gus loved the tech. I have a padded sticker on my backside to keep me from getting bed sores. The surgery took four hours. There were lots and lots of questions. I met my surgeon and two from anesthesiology—one was the nurse anesthetist, and the other was the doctor. I refused a pregnancy test (so silly to ask me at this point in my life) and signed the paper instead.

The last thing I wanted was to panic right before going under. So, when the nurse offered me a Valium, I took it without hesitation. Anything to steady my nerves. I was then wheeled into the operating suite. There were so many people in there: I think there were eight, the breast surgeon, the plastic surgeon, an anesthesiologist, their assistant, and the nursing team. I moved over to the table and got settled. The next thing I knew, the mask was on, and Dr. Johnson was singing me to sleep.[11]

The next memory is waking up in recovery. My chest feels like I did a horribly hard workout. My pecs and armpits hurt. They gave me one OxyContin since I said my pain was an eight out of 10. I slowly woke up and eventually got dressed. They were unsure when I should take my blood thinner, so they held me for a bit until they could leave a message for the doctor.

I got dressed and went to the bathroom. My urine was bright, dark blue! Thank goodness I had been warned at some point. I have no idea how much contrast they put in me to track the lymph nodes. It must have been a lot. I am still noticing blue urine this morning. Claire came for a bit yesterday. It was so good to see her in between the slow blinks.

I don't need narcotics today. I walked Tapi, and she didn't pull at all. I think she sensed I was in pain.

---

[11] She's famous for this here in Portland. She sings all her patients to sleep. I don't remember what she sang during this surgery. When she put my medical port in my chest earlier in the year, she sang "Raindrops on Roses." It was lovely and comforting. And memorable.

I'm going to rest and eat today. I need to walk slowly and breathe in the spirometer to get my lungs back in shape. My throat is very sore from the intubation. Lots of cough drops today, too.

I am so packed with gauze, and so swollen, I can't tell how small my boobs are. It looks the same to me. I will get to unwrap everything tomorrow.

Thank you for all the texts and encouraging notes yesterday. It was helpful. They kept me from running out of the hospital.

I know the doctor spoke to me when I was waking up. I am pretty sure she said everything went well.

We are waiting for pathology to be sure. It can take up to a week. Now for some breakfast.

When the full pathology came back, it was good news. The tumor left after chemo was smaller than what they first found—now about 12 millimeters—and the edges around what was removed were clear. None of the three lymph nodes tested showed cancer. The report confirmed my cancer was estrogen- and HER2-positive, which meant there were strong treatments available going forward. In short, the surgery worked, the cancer was out, and I had a clean starting point for the next phase of treatment.

Day 164: Radiation Prep

Today, they see how long I can hold my breath and tattoo me for radiation. This is the initial consultation. I am waiting for them to return and get me positioned on the hard table. The radiation technician just threw a ton of info at me. Today is about the repeatable and precise placement of my body on the table.

The tattoos are done. I was supposed to have three. I ended up with two since I have a well-placed freckle on one side, which they'll use to orient me in the machine, lining me up with the laser, and my tattoos. The other dot is between my breasts. They are tiny dots. They look like someone gently poked me with a Bic pen, and like you should be able to wash them off. It is a weird way to get my first tattoos. I start radiation next Thursday.

Day 170: Radiation Details

Tomorrow is Thursday, so I will get the added fun of a new infusion. It will be every three weeks for a year on the Kadcyla infusions. I had no idea I would have to do this again.

They haven't told me how many radiation sessions there will be in total. It's every weekday for either 16 or 25 days. I expect to be exhausted by the end of August. I am just going with the flow.

Hoping to go to Boston in September. I am feeling okay after the surgery, but still swollen, and not sleeping well. The adventure continues.

Tapi is still here. No adoption inquiries yet. I may have to take things into my own hands and advertise her online.

I met a friend from Intel for a late coffee. She left last year. I may work on some projects for her new team. I'll be working on a quote tomorrow. That is something to look forward to. Hugs to you all. (Gentle ones)

Day 171: And It Begins...Radiation

It will be 16 sessions. And one is done —15 sessions to go. I'll be done in mid-August. The Chihuahuas are coming tomorrow, so that'll be a good distraction.

I'm doing okay so far. I held my breath for the requisite amount of time while the machine did its work. I'm hoping my heart and lungs come out of this okay. Tapi was happy to see me when I got back. She's a squeaker. Wishing everyone a great weekend.

Day 179: My Baby Turns 20

Happy Friday. Today, I no longer have a teenager. Claire turns 20 at 11:30 pm tonight. Julia came over, and we had brunch to celebrate.

I finished my eighth radiation treatment this afternoon. Halfway mark today. Next week, four in a row. And then the final four the week after.

Other than some exhaustion and dry skin (I am moisturizing a lot), I am weathering it okay so far.

They've decided that I will start taking Tamoxifen daily after this is done. Follow-up appointments with the breast and plastic surgeon are next week. And preparing for an event where I am speaking.

All is well. Headed to the Indiana Jones movie tonight with Gus. And then Blue Öyster Cult this weekend.

Day 185: Tired

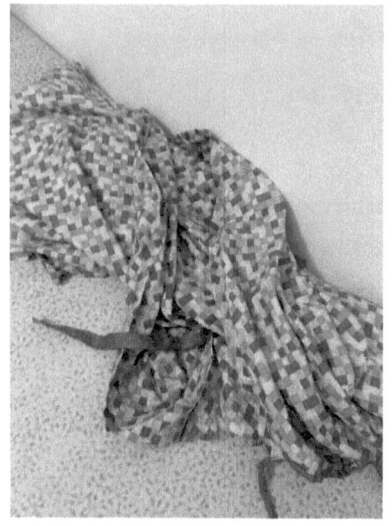

I am so sick and tired of this pattern on the dressing gowns. This is the one I change into for every test, scan, and radiation treatment here at Good Sam.

Four more radiation sessions to go. I am here at the hospital waiting for the doc (weekly check-in), and then I can leave.

They ordered my Tamoxifen, and it should come by mail this week. Next Thursday, I enter the maintenance phase. Infusions every three weeks—a new drug to help with bone loss (Zometa) – and daily Tamoxifen.

Later today, I have my second post-op with the plastic surgeon.

I have a referral for some compression undergarments to help with the edema. I will have to wear a sleeve on planes.[12]

I started specialized (lymphedema-reducing) physical therapy to see if we could get my ears to drain and reduce the swelling under my arms and my trunk. I am less swollen than before, but more swollen than I want to be.

I'm hoping to get released for Pilates and weightlifting today. I need to get back to working out regularly.

---

[12] It turns out I am doing fine on planes. Since my cancer was caught so early and I only had 3 lymph nodes removed, I haven't had any issues with my arm swelling.

Day 189: Almost There!

Today, I watched a woman ring the bell to celebrate her last radiation treatment.

My last one is Thursday at 1:55 pm, then I will ring the bell. Let me know if you want to come. It's in the basement. Parking Lot three. We can get your parking ticket validated.

I neglected to record the details in my diary when the radiation was done. I was so exhausted. The exhaustion is cumulative—building and building and not dissipating until 11 days after the last treatment. Friends came and watched me ring the bell. Julia snuck champagne in, and we had a small toast in the lobby. We also had cupcakes, and we shared the leftovers with the staff. My skin was red and raw, like a severe sunburn, and over the last three days, I developed a rash. Some prescription hydrocortisone cream, three times a day, cleared it up, and the redness faded over the coming weeks—just like a bad sunburn.

Moving On

You've just walked with me through the rawest part of my story: the shock of diagnosis, the grind of treatment, and the messy mix of fear, humor, and hope that carried me through. But when the last infusion is done, and the final radiation beam clicks off, life doesn't simply return to what it was. The truth is that treatment is just one chapter. What follows can be even harder to put into words: the losses that linger, the resilience it takes to rebuild, and the search for a "new normal" that doesn't feel normal at all.

Section Two steps into that space. These essays are less about a medical calendar and more about life itself, identity, strength, and the ways we piece ourselves back together. Think of this as the bridge between my lived story and the practical guidance that comes later. Before we get tactical again, I want to pause on grief—the invisible companion of healing. This part is more emotional than prescriptive, but I'll share what helped me navigate it in real life. My hope is that you'll see pieces of your own experience here and find something steady to hold onto.

SECTION TWO

Life after Treatment

When treatment ends, the story doesn't. What follows is quieter but no less demanding: grief, identity shifts, and the long work of rebuilding. These essays capture the aftershocks of cancer and the resilience required to move forward.

Chapter 6: Loss, Lessons, and Grief

Grief isn't just about losing people—it's also about losing parts of ourselves. Life shifts in ways we never expected, and each change demands a different kind of resilience. Before you keep reading, know that this part of the book shifts gears. It's less about tactics and more about truth— the messy middle between endings and beginnings. I'll still offer small things that helped me cope, but this section lives in the emotional space of loss, where healing first takes root.

If you're in treatment or freshly out of it, these stories might mirror your own losses—physical, emotional, or spiritual. I've added small reflections and practices that helped me make sense of grief when everything felt uncertain. Take what fits; leave what doesn't.

Some losses are like a missed note you barely catch. Others are like a fading refrain, growing softer until it's gone. And then there are the crashing chords—loud, sudden, impossible to ignore—that reverberate through your whole being.

Looking back, I didn't realize it at the time, but the way I coped with my first losses helped prepare me for the bigger ones. This section will explore how grief builds, how it manifests in different ways, and how we move forward, not past it, but with it. When you're in the thick of it, "moving forward" can sound impossible. In the pages ahead, I share how I learned to do it in tiny, uneven steps—sometimes practical, sometimes emotional, always human.

Losing My Dad: The Day Superman Died

I had a weird feeling as I walked down the hall to my desk. I had been working for nearly a year at my first high-tech job out of college, in finance. My soon-to-be husband worked in engineering, just a few rows away. We'd often grab coffee together, a small comfort in the corporate world.

As I walked towards my cubicle, I heard my desk phone ringing. I had changed the ringer so it wouldn't blend in with the others in the row of identical cubicles. That sound—mine, distinct from the rest—sent a wave of unease through me.

I picked up. "Hello?"

"Vikki—it's me, Mena."

It was my dad's wife. She was hysterical. Her words were tangled in sobs, trying to explain in English but failing. My stomach tightened as I felt my heart begin to race. I couldn't understand her, but I could feel it. Something was wrong.

I interrupted. "Mena, should I be sitting down for this conversation?"

"Yes," she said simply.

My pulse pounded. What the hell is happening?

"Tell me in Portuguese," I said.

And then, in a language that felt more familiar, she shattered my world.

"They're hiking in now. To find the plane. Your uncle came down from Rhode Island. He's with the search team."

"Wait, back up. What happened?"

"I think your dad is dead."

I froze. No. That's not possible.

I pressed hold on the beige phone console. My hands shook as I punched the pre-programmed button for Gus's line.

"Gus, I have Mena on the phone. She says she thinks my dad is dead. Something about his plane. Can you come over here?"

I didn't wait for his answer. I clicked back to Mena.

"What happened?"

She told me they had shared a car since they had returned to the U.S. She was at work, expecting him to pick her up at 5 pm, but he didn't show up. This was in 1992, well before cell phones became the norm. She couldn't reach him at home. She was angry, thinking he was distracted and had forgotten her. She caught a ride home with a colleague. He wasn't there either. After remembering his plan for the day, a friend drove her to the small airport where Dad kept his Mooney M20E, a sleek, high-performance plane someone in his circle nicknamed "the Ferrari of the skies."

His car was parked near the hangar, with the sunroof open, and his driving glasses and jacket on the seat. But the plane was gone. Dad had started flying when he and my mom returned from Brazil in 1967. It was right after I was born. He and his best friend, Mark, my godfather, trained together and earned their instrument flight ratings. And he was meticulous when it came to flying: No alcohol within 48 hours of a flight; checklists followed to the letter; everything by the book.

Mom, my sister, and I always thought he was Superman. He could fly planes, race sailboats, and drive fast cars. Even though he was a finance guy, he could fix anything. He also had a need for speed and control.

Superman Doesn't Die—Does He?

My mom once told me about flying with him in a four-seater Cessna when the plane iced over. That's not good since ice adds drag, disrupts airflow, reduces lift, and increases stall speed. At one point in the flight, Dad asked her to point the flashlight at the windscreen. He had realized the entire plane was iced over. There was no panic—just calm directions that she followed as his navigator. He gradually descended until the ice melted and they landed safely.

Life was like that with Dad. There was another time when we were out on his brand-new 40-foot sailboat. The wind was strong, and the waves were high. It was a beautiful sunny day off the coast of Brazil, near Ilha dos Papagaios (Parrot Island). I was up on the bow, watching the waves and looking for dolphins, when he yelled for us to take down the sails. It made no sense—until we realized he had lost control of the helm.

He lifted the tiller right out of the hull to prove his point. It wasn't attached to the rudder anymore. We were headed straight for the island, with the wind in the sails, pushing the boat sideways. We scrambled to get the sails down and slow the boat down. The anchor dragged and eventually caught as we got closer to the uninhabited and very rocky island. We bobbed in the choppy waves and shot off flares until we got the attention of nearby boats. Eventually, we were towed into the yacht club, where we took photos of the broken rudder, and my mom popped a bottle of whiskey open to calm the adults' nerves. Once again, we were safe.

The Things You Can't Control
When Mena got to the airfield, the fence was shut, and she could see the car near the hangar. After checking the car and the hangar, she realized his plane was missing. She deduced that he had thought he'd be right back after testing out the instrument the technician had repaired, so he hadn't bothered to close the sunroof in the Nissan.

The next day, the authorities launched a search-and-rescue operation. They spotted the plane wreckage from the air. A search party gathered, and after hiking in, they found what was left of him. My uncle identified his body. Years later, I requested the autopsy report. No photos—just the cold details. He was missing part of his face and jaw. The coroner's report listed him as six inches shorter than he was in life. The plane was a total loss.

Losing my dad was not my first encounter with grief. I had lost both my grandfathers in the years before that. That was hard. Especially watching my parents lose their dads. However, this was next level. After all, how does Superman die? He had survived so many near misses before. They couldn't figure out what had gone wrong. The FAA collected the wreckage and reconstructed the plane. They autopsied his body. Nothing indicated a problem. They chalked it up to "failure of the pilot to maintain control of the airplane." We couldn't believe it. After years of speaking with experts and Dad's friend, Jim, the only logical and straightforward explanation was that he hit some turbulence, he was knocked out after hitting his head on the side of the plane, and then slumped over his yoke controls and went down at a 70-degree angle into the side of a mountain, as described by an eyewitness.

At 24, I learned that grief isn't linear. It doesn't come in neat, predictable waves. It ambushes you. Some people work through it. Others get stuck. What helped me then was structure: a journal, a morning walk, anything that gave shape to the day. If you're grieving right now, try giving yourself one small anchor—a routine, a sound, or a space that reminds you life still has rhythm.

Losing My Knee Health: A Life Redefined

Cancer wasn't my first health crisis. Long before my diagnosis, my body had already forced me to redefine what resilience meant. My dad died in 1992—the year after I started my first job in Finance at Intel—and nearly two decades later, in 2009, a horrific soccer accident changed my life again. Those two events taught me different lessons about grief, recovery, and adapting when life doesn't go as planned. Before I ever faced cancer, I'd already learned what it meant to live with a new reality.

February 6, 2009, 9:30 PM

Some dates become markers, dividing life into before and after. For me, this was one of those moments. Before that night, I was able-bodied. After that night, I wasn't. I didn't know it then, but this wasn't just an injury; it was the beginning of an entirely new way of moving through the world.

I grew up in Brazil, where soccer, known as *futebol* to Brazilians, was everything. I fell in love with the game early, and for 31 years, I played as a goalie. If you've met me, you might find that funny. I'm 5'3" on a good day, and most goalkeepers tower over me. But I didn't care. The thrill of the game, the strategy, and the challenge all fueled me.

Living in Oregon, married with two children, and 44 years old, I was still playing soccer. I had been playing regularly for two years on an all-women's outdoor team before the accident. When the season ended in late 2008, we decided to move indoors. American indoor soccer is nothing like the *Futebol de Salão* I grew up with in Brazil. In the U.S., it's played on a hockey rink covered in carpet, with walls you can bounce the ball off of. It is soccer mixed with basketball rebounds and billiards angles.

During a game that night, my defense lagged behind, leaving me vulnerable. I charged forward to stop an advancing striker. As I planted my left foot and reached for the ball with my hands, she slammed into my left thigh. Hard.

The next thing I knew, I was on my right side, screaming in agony, and clutching my left leg.

Everything was wrong. My body knew it before my brain did.

Women surrounded me immediately—one holding my head, two grasping my hands, and others supporting my leg. Someone asked me for the passcode to my BlackBerry and called my husband to meet me at the hospital. The ambulance arrived, and they gave me as much pain medication as the law allowed before taking me to St. Vincent's Hospital.

The Diagnosis

X-rays confirmed what my body already suspected:

- A dislocated tibia and fibula from my knee.
- I had probably torn every ligament.
- Possible nerve damage.

The doctors weren't sure if I'd ever fully recover—or if I'd even walk normally again.

While I was under sedation, a team of five men relocated the bones after a couple of tries. My husband, tasked with keeping me from instinctively punching anyone, held me in a bear hug as they worked.

I needed surgery. But it was Friday night, and the swelling was too severe. They kept me in the hospital for the weekend, hoping to bring the inflammation down before operating on Monday. When I finally met the surgeon, a giant Canadian orthopedic specialist, just minutes before they put me under, he had a look on his face that I'll never forget, somber and uncertain. "I'll do the best I can," he told me.

The Road to Recovery

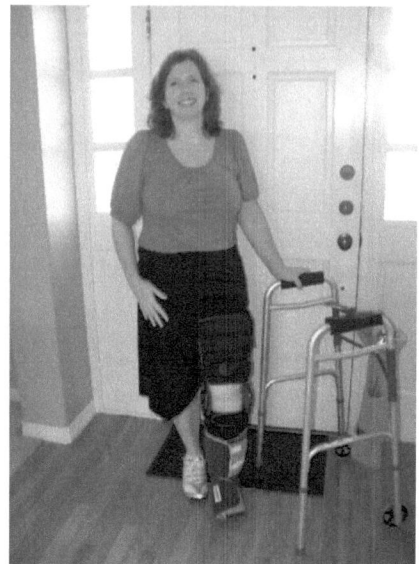

After surgery, they sent me home with a massive immobilizing brace and strict orders: Do not take it off under any circumstances. And do not let your toes touch the ground. I was on heavy painkillers and had to figure out how to navigate daily life in a two-story house with showers upstairs.

My husband, ever the engineer, sprang into action. He secured a shower chair, a waterproof leg cover, a wheelchair, a walker with a tray, and a backpack for carrying essentials. He even wrapped pipe insulation around my crutches to keep my hands from blistering.

Support poured in. Friends brought meals, ran errands, picked up the kids, and kept me company. My sister left her own family for two weeks to help mine adjust. My daughters, only nine and six at the time, stepped up, learning to cook, do laundry, and take care of things around the house.

Learning to Walk Again

In late 2009, after three surgeries, my brain and my right leg didn't trust my left leg anymore. No matter how much I willed it to move, it would not budge. I spent an entire hour just trying to free-stand on my left leg 12 weeks after the third surgery. I couldn't do it. My right leg instinctively wouldn't come off the floor.

My sports medicine physical therapist told me I had to move

into the pool, where the water could take some weight off my legs. Pool therapy helped immediately. I went back to my original PT at the hospital after just three pool therapy sessions.

After graduating from physical therapy, I began working with Sam, a personal trainer who viewed my injury as a challenge, and he customized a rehabilitation program for me. He had me learning how to log-roll my body, crawl, walk over hurdles, practice stairs, and sit and stand as if I were getting in and out of a car. Every movement that had once been effortless had to be learned again, so I wouldn't limp permanently. A few of the muscles in my left leg don't work due to the peroneal nerve damage and ensuing foot drop. I've worked hard to overcome my disability and walk nearly perfectly with an ankle-foot orthosis (brace). I am proud of my accomplishments and grateful to Sam for his guidance and perseverance to help me walk as normally as possible. As I continued to rehabilitate, my doctors wanted my knee to bend more. It was stuck with adhesions from the surgery, and I couldn't bend enough to pedal the recumbent bike.

Trying New Things

I sat and cried in frustration, pain, and anger as I tried to make the complete revolution on the bike in our family room. Even going backwards wasn't working. With the kids in bed, sitting on the bike, tears and snot streaming down my face, Gus approached me with a roll of toilet paper he had snagged from the bathroom. As I tried to wipe my tears and blow my nose, he gently started asking me questions. Typical engineer, and precisely what I needed at that moment. He was going to figure out what I had tried, what wasn't working, and what I hadn't tried yet. The doctor had cautioned me that he might have to put me under anesthesia again to break the adhesions and scar tissue in my knee. I knew I couldn't face another surgery. I was scared. As Gus got to asking me what I hadn't tried, I blurted out 'deep tissue massage therapy'. He asked me why I hadn't done it yet. I said because 'it's going to hurt!' He then asked which was the lesser of two evils: surgery or massage therapy. I told him I'd rather be aware of what was happening, so I chose massage therapy. He asked me what steps I would take the next day. I said I would call Jodie, the massage therapist at the chiropractor's office, and book an appointment.

It ended up taking three appointments. Jodie booked me at the end of the day so I could swear as much as I wanted to without disturbing (or scaring) other people in the other treatment rooms. She asked me to drink lots of water and take some Tylenol before my sessions. I cried a lot during the first two, fists balled up in the sheets, and trying to maintain my sense of humor as she dug deep into every muscle, every tendon, and every sore spot in my battered and scarred knee and leg. She got more movement in each and every session. That third session did the trick. She got it loose enough that I passed the flexion test at my next physical therapy appointment and avoided surgery. I am forever grateful to her for helping me avoid manual manipulation under anesthesia.

Realizing I'll Never Be Normal Again

Four years after my recovery from the soccer accident, I was doing a side shuffle in the gym, and I twisted my left ankle when my sneaker got caught between two rubber floor mats. Down I went. I realized I had done some damage when I couldn't stand up. I had popped the patellar tendon right off the bone. I had surgery a few days later and then got busy with physical therapy and rehabilitation. I went back to my trainer, Sam, and got additional support. The recovery was relatively fast—I knew what I was doing. However, if I sat too long, things would tighten up and become sore and stiff.

It was hard to walk at the end of the day after sitting at my desk.

One evening, after a long workday, I was limping down the long hallway to go home when a woman I barely knew stopped me. "What's wrong with you?" she asked. "Why are you limping so badly? Why aren't you better yet?" Her words didn't sound like curiosity; it felt like an accusation, as if I hadn't worked hard enough to get "back to normal."

I was stunned, tired, and angry. Usually, I am comfortable when people ask about my injury. My brace was visible when I wore skirts in the summer, and I didn't mind explaining. But this was different. This was someone telling me that my progress wasn't good enough. The truth was, I would never be "better." I would never be back to the person I had been before the injury. And eventually, I had to make peace with that.

Lessons I Carry Forward

If what you're doing isn't working, stop and try something new.

Lean on the experts and those who know how to do what you need done.

Health insurance shouldn't be a privilege: it's a necessity.

Slow down and enjoy the journey. When you move more slowly, you see more.

No matter how challenging, look for the silver linings. There will be things to be grateful for every day. Those lessons weren't abstract. I wrote them down, taped them to my bathroom mirror, and revisited them whenever I forgot what progress looked like. If you're keeping a notebook through treatment, leave a few pages after each section to jot down your own lessons—you'll be amazed how your perspective shifts over time.

What Loss Teaches Us about Living

My knee injury forced me to redefine myself. It took something from me, yet it gave me perspective. I learned that living isn't just about healing, it's also about adapting. Adapting starts small: a stretch instead of a run, a shorter workday, asking for help instead of pushing through. The adjustments are the work. Write down one area where you're adapting right now—it might not feel like progress, but it is.

That's how I found my way to fencing. For years, I had been the mom on the sidelines, fetching water, checking schedules, and cheering on my daughter, Julia. One day, a fellow fencer suggested I try wheelchair fencing. I had no idea you didn't have to use a wheelchair every day to qualify—you merely had to have permanent nerve damage that made able-bodied fencing impossible.

What began as curiosity turned into training, competing, and eventually traveling with the U.S. team. It entertained me, gave me back a sense of competition, and showed me that I could still live life to the fullest—even with a nerve-damaged leg. I even came within six points of making the U.S. Paralympic Team for Rio in 2016. To qualify, I would have had to take first place at the final tournament. Instead, I finished second. And while that result kept me off the team, it brought me a different kind of victory: I beat the Brazilian fencer on her home turf in São Paulo. I lost to a younger, more seasoned fencer from my own team. Missing Rio by six points could have felt like failure, but instead it became proof that I belonged on that stage at all. That knowledge stayed with me long after the medals were handed out.

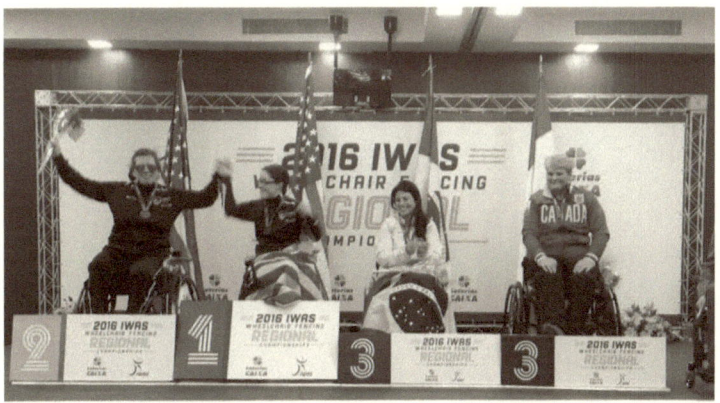

Years later, when cancer came for me, I realized something: I had been here before. I had already faced losing control of my body. That first doctor wasn't sure I would walk again. I had already learned what it means to fight through recovery. And I had already seen how much support from your family, friends, and the medical professionals matters.

Even so, nothing could have fully prepared me for what was coming. I carried those earlier lessons into cancer without realizing it. They became the survival tools I didn't know I had—proof that resilience is cumulative. Every hardship teaches something you'll need later.

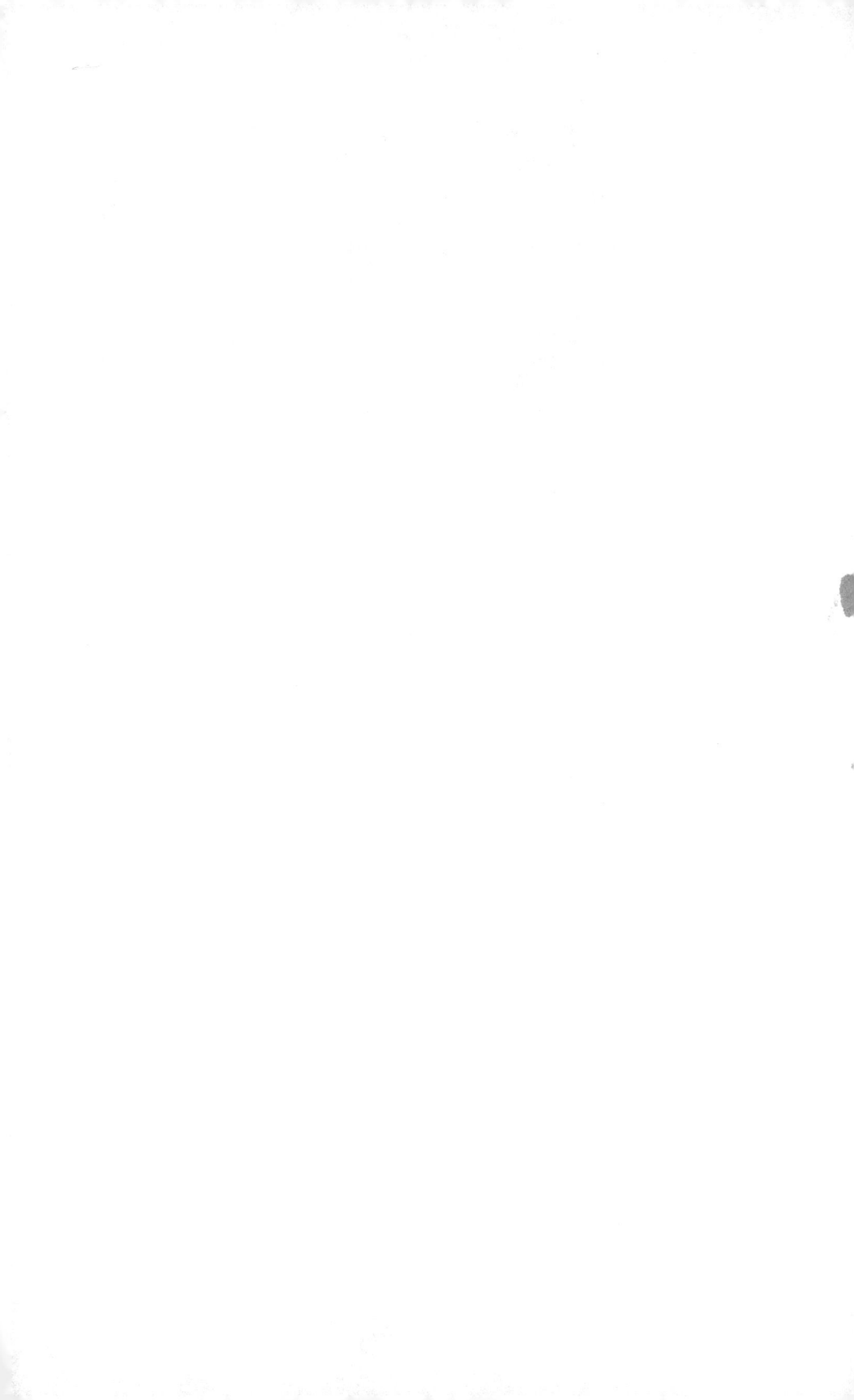

Chapter 7: Losing Control: Panic Attacks and Body Functions

I have always thought of myself as strong, capable, and resilient—someone who could face challenges head-on, even when they seemed insurmountable. But at the beginning of my cancer journey, all that self-assurance crumbled. I had my first-ever panic attack, and it was like nothing I had ever experienced before.

The Panic Attack

I collapsed in a heap, sobbing uncontrollably. Not the quiet, restrained crying that you can stifle after a few deep breaths, but the kind of raw, gut-wrenching sobs that leave you shaking and gasping for air. It felt like part of me floated up and was watching this broken, panicking version of myself unravel. I could not stop it. I couldn't control the flood of emotions, fear, despair, embarrassment, depression, and, above all, the overwhelming sense of losing control.

We were waiting for the results of my breast biopsy. Everything was too unknown, and my mind could not find a path forward. I could not see a way out. Gus had to call for help, and we got a prescription for Valium to help calm me down. Even that bugged me—that I had to medicate myself to handle what was happening. That was not me! I was supposed to be strong and capable, yet here I was, reduced to a sobbing, shaking wreck.

Gus drove me to the pharmacy because I couldn't function. I cried so hard that I gave myself the hiccups. I could not believe this was happening to me. If you had asked me what I most feared in life, I would have said losing control—control over my life, my body, or my choices. And now, what I feared most was happening in real time.

At that moment, I had no choice but to surrender. I had to jump in the boat, let go of the oars, and trust the doctors, nurses, and medical team to steer me to the correct destination: being declared cancer-free.

It was the hardest thing I have ever done, but also a turning point. Surrendering doesn't mean giving up: it means finding strength in letting others help you navigate when the waters are too rough to manage alone.

I return to resilience practices in Chapter 27, which helped me regain my footing.

Pooping My Pants on Camera

I have been on camera more times than I can count. Large auditoriums, global conferences, Zoom calls, you name it. I don't get stage fright anymore. But nothing—absolutely nothing—could have prepared me for what happened that day.

COVID made virtual meetings a necessity—for staff meetings, for connecting with my teammates over coffee a few times a week, and for presenting at conferences that suddenly went online. I have been recorded inside large auditoriums, with people watching from desks and viewing rooms around the world. Being on camera is something I am mostly comfortable with. So, when a company asked me to have a live, on-camera conversation from my house during chemo, I thought, *Sure!*

I'll be at home. Maybe the wig won't be as obvious over Zoom. I'll be talking about a topic I love, and the other person is an expert, very comfortable on camera, too. It'll be fine. I'll be fine. I might even have some fun sharing insights and answering audience questions.

It had to be more fun than rotting on my couch in between chemo sessions.

I had been out in the car a few times before the on-camera conversation. I didn't venture far because when my gastrointestinal tract was ready to purge, it didn't leave me a lot of time to find the nearest bathroom. The diarrhea was relentless, immediate, and non-negotiable.

Once, I ventured up to the supermarket. It's about two miles from my house, a seven-minute drive. That day, I got in the car and was about halfway home when I knew. I wasn't going to make it. My stomach clenched. My body had decided it was time. *Oh God.* I called Gus.

"Hey, can you open the garage door, open the door to the house, corral Dakota so he doesn't wander off, and come outside?"

"What's wrong?" he asked.

"I'm having a bathroom emergency. I need the fastest and clearest path to the bathroom, and I have groceries in the car. I won't have time to even turn off the car. I need to park and run."

Being the amazing human he is, he cleared a path for me, and I whizzed by him, making it to the bathroom in the nick of time. It was insane. I told my sister about it later, and she recommended I wear adult diapers on my next trip out of the house. I wasn't sure I'd ever leave the house again, except for chemo or a doctor's appointment.

Later, I was on Reddit and saw a woman vulnerably write about her recent trip to the grocery store. She had walked there. She didn't have a car. And she did poop her pants as she walked home. She was ashamed. Horrified. People on the street could tell. She said it was the lowest point of her treatment.

I thought I could empathize. *No, not yet.*

My full-on empathy came a few weeks later, on camera, in the middle of a live conversation. Mid-sentence, I felt it. *No.*

No, no, no. Not now. Not on camera. Not in front of a live audience. My body didn't care.

I fought to keep my face neutral, my voice steady, and my smile intact. No one had a clue. Inside, I was unraveling. I realized that my body wasn't going to wait, and with a smile on my face, still speaking, I proceeded to poop my pants. I sat in the mess for 15 minutes until the recording finished and the call ended. Then I walked to the kitchen, got a garbage bag, went into the bathroom, stripped everything I was wearing into the bag, and after cleaning up the best I could, hopped in the shower.

What an experience. As I scrubbed the chair I had been sitting in for the recording, I tried to focus on gratitude. *What was I grateful for?* The fact that I hadn't been in my car. That I hadn't been walking a long way from my house. That my husband had been out of the house. That no one had a clue what I was going through on the video call. That I hadn't been in an auditorium in front of 350 people, having to excuse myself to go to the bathroom. And that I didn't have to tell anyone.

It was awful. It was humiliating. But it was... survivable. And if I could survive *that*, I could survive anything. That experience taught me that surviving isn't about dignity—it's about endurance. When the worst happens, look for one small reason to be grateful; it breaks shame's grip just enough to let resilience back in.

Then I popped some more Imodium and took a nap.

Later, when I told a close friend what had happened, I expected pity or embarrassment on my behalf. Instead, she laughed—a deep, belly laugh. And then I laughed, too. Hard. Because sometimes, when the worst thing happens, and you come out on the other side, all you can do is laugh. It wasn't just about surviving the moment. It was about realizing that, even in the messiest, most humiliating experiences, I was still *me*. Still strong. Still whole. And still here.

Grief, Loss, and Moving Forward

Grief isn't something you just move on from—it's something you move forward with. It's the shadow of love, the proof that something mattered. You grieve because you loved your old self, your loved one, your job, or the life you thought you'd have. Instead of trying to push grief away, I've learned to carry it with me, to honor it, and to let it be a reminder of the deep connections and experiences that shaped me.

Understanding the stages of grief doesn't mean you follow them in order. Grief is messy. It circles back on itself. The key is recognizing where you are and giving yourself the grace to feel it fully. I encourage you to 'name it to tame it.' Be conscious of what you're feeling so you can feel it fully and move forward. When I caught myself spiraling, I used a simple practice: I'd write down the feeling and one sentence about why it was there. Seeing it on paper took some of its power away.

The Seven Stages of Grief
1. Shock & Denial
2. Pain & Guilt
3. Anger & Bargaining
4. Depression, Reflection, Loneliness
5. The Upward Turn
6. Reconstruction & Working Through
7. Acceptance & Hope

Reflection Prompt
Which of these stages feels closest to where you are right now? What does "forward" look like today, even if it's only a breath or a step?

I find the seven stages more complete and more descriptive of what the process of grief really entails. I knew I might bounce between these stages while also helping others find their next steps. But there were things I wasn't prepared for that surprised me. Reflecting on them now, I want to document these insights for anyone going through something similar.

My knee injury and cancer both followed an eerily similar cycle: Shock. Denial. Anger. Grief. Acceptance. Adaptation.

I mourned my mobility. I mourned my hair. I mourned the ease of existing in a body that had once felt like home.

But in both cases, I adapted. I didn't do this by returning to who I was before, but by stepping into who I had become.

Lessons from Pain

When I shattered my leg in 2009, it felt like my life had split into before and after. One moment, I was strong and capable; the next, I was struggling to walk and grappling with a body that no longer worked as I expected it to.

I thought that was the hardest thing I would ever endure.

And then came cancer.

Both experiences redefined me in ways I never anticipated. They forced me to confront loss, resilience, and what it means to keep going when your body feels like it belongs to a stranger. But while they shared common threads, the differences between them were just as profound.

Adaptation and the Long Road to Acceptance
Both recoveries came with pain, physical and emotional.

My knee injury left me with permanent foot drop, a daily reminder that some damage can't be undone. I had to relearn movement, find new ways to navigate the world, and accept that my body had limits I never expected. And to wear a brace every day, most days fighting to get my toes in without one or two curling under my foot.

Cancer's aftermath was more insidious. The fatigue, the nerve pain, the loss of feeling in my toes on my good side, the scars—these were things no one had prepared me for. Unlike my knee, where the worst was front-loaded, my cancer recovery stretched on, unpredictable and endless. There was no finish line—no moment when I felt I could declare myself healed.

The Differences That Made All the Difference

For all their similarities, my injury and cancer experience were worlds apart. The biggest difference? Cancer didn't end when treatment did.

My knee injury was a moment: a single traumatic event with a long, arduous, but ultimately linear recovery. Once I adjusted, it was over.

The cancer never really ended. Treatment may have finished, but the specter of recurrence lingers. There is no clean break, no true "after." Even in remission, cancer is a shadow that never fully disappears.

The treatment for my knee ended, but the result of the injury stayed with me, visible to the world in a way that cancer was not. People could see the brace, the limp, and the effort. It made sense to most of them.

Cancer was trickier. In some ways, it was obvious—chemo took my hair, and surgeries left scars—but the worst of it was hidden. What people didn't see: the exhaustion so profound I could barely stand, the neuropathy that made every step uncertain, the emotional weight I carried long after treatment ended. Just because I looked "okay" didn't mean I was.

The biggest difference between my knee injury and cancer was how people treated me. When you have a physical injury, people respond with sympathy. They offer to carry things, hold doors open, and acknowledge the difficulty.

Cancer elicits something different: pity, fear, and even avoidance. Some people say too much, while some say nothing at all. And the word "brave" gets thrown around, even when you don't feel brave. Bravery became an expectation, not a choice. No one called me brave for learning to walk again after my knee injury. But cancer? The moment I lost my hair, bravery was assigned to me, whether I felt it or not.

Cancer also weighs differently on you mentally than an injury, even a serious injury, does. There was no moment in my knee recovery where I thought, "*Will this kill me?*"

Reflection Prompt
If this is where you are—wondering how to trust your body again—try naming one thing your body still does for you: breathing, walking, digesting, healing from a paper cut. Gratitude for the smallest function can rebuild faith in the body you inhabit.

With cancer, I wasn't just healing. I was fighting my own body, unsure if I could trust it again. I was waiting for test results, facing mortality, and undergoing treatments designed to destroy part of you in the hopes of saving the rest. There is a weight to that: a trauma that lingers in ways an injury never could.

With my knee, the goal for treatment was simple: regain function. Learn to live as normally as possible.

With cancer, the goal was just to live. To exist. To make it through. And once I did, I had to figure out what living even means.

Recovery meant regaining function. Living meant learning to exist in an unfamiliar body and navigating an uncertain future.

Both experiences tested me. Both changed me. But cancer didn't just ask me to recover—it forced me to reimagine my future. It took more than my health; it took certainty, security, and parts of my identity that I am still reclaiming.

And yet, in both cases, I found resilience. I adapted. I kept going. Because what else do you do when your body betrays you? You learn. You adjust. And, somehow, you move forward.

Living isn't about returning to what was. It's about redefining yourself and the road ahead. The scars remain, and so do I – living in a form both altered and renewed. If you're here now—somewhere between loss and rebuilding—these are the things that helped me take my first steps forward.

Putting It Into Practice: Living with Loss

Here are a few things that helped me cope and move forward. I hope that one of these practices helps you.

- Write a short letter to your pre-diagnosis self: tell yourself what you've learned from the journey.

- Ask someone close, "Can you just listen for a few minutes?"

- Create a ritual of release: walk, journal, play a song, or light a candle. You might also write down something you want to move on from, then burn it safely in the fireplace or trash can.

- List one small joy or comfort you can return to each week.

- Allow tears, rest, and silence; they're all forms of healing.

Loss remade me, but it also cleared space for what came next. In the next chapter, I'll share what rebuilding looked like: the mindset, movement, and moments that helped me start again. The practical work of rebuilding begins next.

Chapter 8: Resilience & Rebuilding Identity

Resilience isn't about bouncing back to who you were before; it's about reshaping yourself to fit your new reality.

The Myths of Strength and Resilience

During my breast cancer journey—and even earlier, after my 2009 soccer accident—I realized that when people called me "strong," a "warrior," or a "badass," it was not really about me. It was about them. It reflected their fears and hope that, if they were faced with something similar, they could be as strong as I seemed to be.

The truth is, no one sees us at our worst moments. They do not see the breakdowns, the tears, or the times when we want to give up. They see glimpses of our lives and form their opinions based on those. Strength is not about never breaking—it is about continuing to show up, even when every part of you wants to quit.

Resilience is not something we are born with; it's something we cultivate. It is a skill, a behavior, or a muscle that grows stronger with practice.

I share resilience-building practices you can try yourself in Chapter 27.

The Practice of Self-Forgiveness

One of the most important lessons I have learned is to forgive myself for not being able to do everything, for needing help, or for having bad days. I have had to remind myself to talk to myself the way I'd talk to my best friend, with kindness and compassion.

Resilience is not about never falling down. It is about learning how to get back up, even if it's slower or harder than before. These practices, like muscles, grow stronger the more you use them. They have helped me to build a life focused on healing, strength, and joy.

Adjusting to Big Changes

Recovering from cancer isn't just about physical healing; it's also a journey of coming to terms with all the changes, visible and invisible, that treatment brings. One of the most noticeable changes for many people is hair loss and regrowth. While some might celebrate the return of hair as a symbol of recovery, it is a complex emotional experience for others.

Chemo changed my body in ways I expected—like fatigue and nausea—but some changes still caught me off guard. My hair started growing back before chemo ended; it was gray and dark brown, wiry, and unfamiliar. It felt like my body had aged faster than my mind.

Chemo didn't just change my hair—it changed my whole body. I lost muscle, gained weight, and ate my way through treatment. I placed a weekly Target pickup order, mostly filled with comfort snacks: Pringles, gummy bears, flavored almonds, and chocolate.

While resilience and self-advocacy helped me feel a sense of control, nothing could fully prepare me for the reality of treatment. Chemotherapy, radiation, and the emotional weight of a cancer diagnosis came with unexpected challenges that tested my strength in ways I never anticipated.

Finding Strength in Movement

My journey with fitness has been defined by adaptation and resilience. It began long before my cancer diagnosis, rooted in the serious soccer injury that significantly altered my physical capabilities. Doctors advised me against running or any exercise involving twisting or lateral stress on my rebuilt knee, effectively ruling out many sports I loved. My initial recovery involved extensive physical therapy, followed by working with my trainer, Sam, to relearn how to walk without a limp. We progressed to CrossFit-style workouts, which were effective for a time. However, in 2013, another injury—twisting my ankle and popping my patellar tendon—forced me to re-evaluate my exercise routines. CrossFit, with its higher-impact movements, felt increasingly risky as I aged.

Returning to the gym after that second rehabilitation was challenging. Sam had moved on, needing a job with insurance for his growing family. I felt lost, experimenting with various activities like gym workouts, yoga, parafencing, and walking. Yoga proved particularly frustrating. I spent more time positioning my dysfunctional foot than actually exercising, leaving me feeling defeated. My balance was poor, and I wasn't seeing improvements.

Then, in early 2017, a targeted Facebook advertisement for Pilates appeared. With little knowledge of it, but drawn by the offer of a free session, I signed up. I was hooked from that first session. Reformer Pilates, with its straps, bands, and yoga blocks, allowed me to modify almost any movement to accommodate my foot drop. Unlike yoga, I could fully participate without feeling self-conscious or different. I grew stronger and leaner, even losing weight. This success was a turning point, motivating me to find a new gym and a trainer, eventually leading me to Brett, with whom I've worked consistently for most of the past seven years (with a break during COVID).

Pilates became my foundation, providing a low impact, yet effective way to build strength and improve mobility, both before and after my cancer diagnosis. After I was diagnosed and throughout my treatment (chemo, surgery, and radiation), I prioritized staying healthy and avoiding germs. This meant taking a break from both Pilates and the gym. I focused on nutrition—protein shakes, protein-rich meals, and supplements approved by the cancer-medication pharmacist—to support my body.

As the radiation-induced exhaustion began to lift, I was eager to return to movement. Thankfully, I had maintained my Pilates studio membership. I knew I needed to start slowly, so I began with Level 1 classes every other day. The results were immediate and profound. I felt like the Tin Man after being oiled—stiff joints started to move freely again. On days without Pilates, the contrast was stark: I felt stiff, awkward, and unmotivated. I quickly ramped up my practice, eventually attending classes six days a week, and now seven. I have also returned to level 2 classes.

I attend a 6:00 a.m. class during the week, an 8:30 a.m. class on Saturdays, and a 7:00 a.m. class on Sundays. This routine has become essential. While it might seem excessive, the Tamoxifen I take depletes my body of crucial elements like bone-supporting minerals, estrogen, and progesterone. These hormones lubricate the joints, and their absence leads to significant stiffness. Starting my day with Pilates helps me move more easily, become more flexible, and stay pain-free. Beyond the physical benefits, it provides crucial mental grounding. For those 50 minutes, I disconnect from everything else, focusing on instructions, mindful body awareness, and allowing the stresses of daily life to fade away.

However, I also understood that Pilates alone wasn't enough, particularly after my cancer experience. A worrying side effect of chemotherapy and hormone therapy is osteoporosis, and my bone scan confirmed I had progressed directly to this condition, skipping osteopenia. This was a wake-up call. Current research suggests that weight-bearing exercise is crucial, and, specifically, being able to perform a Farmer's Carry is a good indicator of strength and bone health.

Therefore, I incorporated weightlifting into my routine three days a week, working with Brett. He changes up my workout every 12 weeks, and I do it all, including pushing, pulling, glute, and leg exercises. We also incorporate functional movements like push-ups, step-ups, and pull-ups. I also aim to walk five to six days a week, wearing my weighted vest to further stimulate bone growth. I've received three Zometa infusions to aid bone regeneration. I maintain a diet rich in green vegetables and take Vitamin D supplements.

Another challenge I faced was neuropathy from the Kadcyla, resulting in a loss of sensation in a few toes on my "good" side. This initially caused significant balance issues. I sought help from a neurological physical therapist, Abby, who was incredible. She assessed my capabilities and designed exercises to refine my motor skills, enhancing my balance and stability. These exercises, combined with Brett's focus on strengthening my left hamstring and stabilizing my left knee, have led to significant improvement. I now walk with greater confidence and a longer stride.

Weightlifting, like Pilates, has become more than just physical exercise. It has restored my confidence and a sense of power in my body. A few months ago, I reached a point where I could leg-press Brett—a fun, tangible demonstration of my regained strength. He climbed up on the press instead of the weighted plates, and I completed 15 reps.

Being strong encompasses both physical and mental fortitude. Exercise, with its demand for mindful attention and consistent effort, strengthens both the body and the mind. I've become more resilient, recognizing my capabilities through hard work and focus. Finding enjoyment and setting goals within my workouts is crucial. Brett keeps me entertained and helps me build the body that will support me through this next chapter of life, a chapter I hope to enter strong, healthy, and capable of power walking well into my 90s. Weightlifting reminds me that strength is not just about muscles—it's about identity, confidence, and how we carry ourselves. That lesson became even more important once cancer forced me to confront the loss of something tied so deeply to identity: my hair.

Chapter 9: Leaning Into Gratitude for Your Body

Cancer changes your body in ways you can't always prepare for. Scars, acne, hair loss, weight changes, loss of appetite, and taste buds don't work correctly—all of it can feel like a series of losses stacked on top of each other. You look in the mirror and sometimes don't recognize yourself. It takes time to process those changes and time to find ways to love yourself again.

One of the most important lessons I learned was to take pride in the body that endured so much. This body carried me through months of chemo, surgery, and radiation. This body endured needles, a medicine port, blood draws, heavy-duty drugs, and the relentless cycle of fatigue and recovery. This body is carrying me forward now, even after everything it has been through. Even when it felt unfamiliar, it was still mine, still trying, still working in the background to heal.

In Pilates, instructors often close class by saying, *"Thank your body for what it could do today."* That line has stayed with me. It's simple, but powerful. It reminds me that gratitude isn't about what I wish my body could do, but about honoring what it managed in that moment. Some days, that meant something as small as making it to the shower, keeping food down, or finally falling asleep. Other days, I was grateful the anti-diarrhea drugs worked so I could sit through dinner without rushing away, or even enjoy a concert without worry. Later, I celebrated when food started tasting right again, when flavors came back, and meals felt like pleasure instead of fuel.

There were even unexpected gifts. My rosacea, something I had struggled with for years, cleared up during chemo. It was strange to be thankful for a skin condition disappearing in the middle of something so brutal, but it was a gift nonetheless. And when my hair came back, I got to experience curls for the first time in my life. They were wild, unexpected curls—ones I didn't quite love, but I tried to embrace them as part of this temporary, shifting version of me. These weren't dramatic miracles. They were small, ordinary surprises that made me pause, smile, and remember that, even in the hardest seasons, life can hand you something different —something good. That's the power of a gratitude practice. Some people use journals and write down three things they're grateful for each day. They don't have to be big or profound—in fact, the smaller the better. A cup of coffee that tastes just right. A good laugh with a friend. A nap that leaves you feeling almost human again. A beautiful sunrise. A walk through the trees with your dog. If you chase those three things every day, they begin to add up. Over time, the practice builds a kind of muscle memory for noticing what's right instead of only what's wrong.

And don't forget to include your body in that gratitude. This is the body that held you through the worst of it. It may be scarred, it may feel different, but it's still yours. Thank it for carrying you to treatment, for taking in medicine, for absorbing rest, for showing up for you again and again. Gratitude doesn't erase the pain or the losses, but it helps shift the story from *my body is failing me* to *my body is still here, doing its best to carry me.*

That mindshift is everything.

I expand on Pilates, weightlifting, and physical resilience later in the Physical Strength section.

Reflection Prompt

Take a few minutes to name three things you're grateful for today. At least one of them should be something your body managed—no matter how small. Maybe it was climbing the stairs, laughing until your stomach hurt, tasting food the way it used to taste, or simply getting through another infusion. Write them down, or say them out loud. Notice how it feels to shift from what's wrong to what's still right.

Physical Changes and Coping

Even though I didn't cry at the time, losing my hair was the most challenging part for me. Maybe it's because of my childhood and some experiences I had after getting a short haircut and being misgendered. Those in Generation X will remember the "Dorothy Hamill" haircut. Claire, my younger daughter, recently found a photo of me from that time and said I looked like a boy with that haircut. Perhaps it's something else. I'd love to say that how my hair looks doesn't matter to me, but it wouldn't be true.

Looking like myself—with bangs and long hair—has always mattered to me.

Dealing with nausea, diarrhea, vomiting, lethargy, and everything else treatment threw at me was somehow easier than losing my hair. Maybe that makes me vain—or perhaps it just means my identity is tied to how I see myself in the mirror. I'm still not sure why it hit so hard. But it did.

For some, hair loss might not be a big deal. Some women describe losing their hair as freeing. For me, it wasn't freeing. It felt like I was losing myself. We all have different grief points.

When I had surgery to remove my gallbladder at nineteen, laparoscopic techniques weren't common yet. I came out with a 12-inch scar across my abdomen. I didn't look at it or acknowledge it as part of me for years. The idea that someone had their hands inside my body—and that my body now carried a permanent reminder—disturbed me deeply.

Today, my hair is shoulder-length again. When I catch my reflection, I smile. There was a time I avoided my own gaze. Now, I recognize myself again—changed, but still here.

I gained a lot of weight during treatment. When "chemo brain" hit me full force, I lost my ability to hold high-level conversations. But even then, none of that bothered me as much as losing my hair.

It took about 18 months for me to feel like myself again. After radiation, I returned to the Pilates studio. I also returned to weightlifting. Not only does weight-lifting challenge me physically, but it should also help reverse the damage done to my bones by the cancer treatment. At this point, I've dropped about thirty pounds, and I feel strong.

One thing I've learned along the way is to be patient and kind to myself. As a "Type A" personality, I have always driven myself to do more, be better, and deliver results faster. This self-imposed pressure was not helpful or necessary during my medical journey. I learned to talk to myself the way I'd talk to my best friend—with encouragement, compassion, and love.

Thoughts on the Warrior Trope

I am not a fan of the warrior language and the pink ribbons, t-shirts, and tchotchkes that surround breast cancer patients. I used to like the color pink. Now it feels like a reminder of the most unpleasant parts of the journey I was on in 2023. I had issues throughout the year with the word *fight* as well. It implies that, if you do not survive, you may not have done it right or worked hard enough to recover, which is profoundly unfair to those who lose their lives to this disease. They fought in their own way, just as I and many others have fought before me.

I have thought a lot about how we're treated for breast cancer—poisoning our bodies, cutting out tumors and tissue, and then burning what's left to catch anything that might have been missed. It is medieval. All of this happens after our breasts are squeezed like pancakes during a mammogram, probed during an ultrasound, and photographed while dangling naked during an MRI.

There has to be a better way. Testing and treatment have come a long way, and I am grateful for the advances, but the process is still brutal. One in eight women goes through this, and, for those with more advanced breast cancer, the treatment never ends. They spend their lives in a cycle of chemo, radiation, and surgeries to prolong their time with loved ones. It is heroic, but it's also horrific.

We need to do better. We need to fund more breast cancer research. We need to support the women in our lives who are suffering through treatment. And we need to redefine what it means to be strong.

Strength does not have to look like standing up, yelling, or educating everyone. Strength can be a quiet statement on a t-shirt. It can be as simple as showing up for your appointments. It can be putting one foot in front of the other when you feel like you cannot. Or it can be planning how you will get through the next hour as you sit on the toilet and everything you've ever eaten seems to pour out of you.

It is okay to cry. It is OK to rail against the system, the disease, and the unfairness of it all. I did all of that. I yelled. I cried. I swore I was not getting out of bed ever again— though my bladder and bowels quickly reminded me that I didn't have that option. I lived on my couch for 12 weeks, unable to do the simplest tasks, like laundry or unloading the dishwasher. Luckily for Gus and me, we have a lot of underwear.

Forgive yourself for what you cannot do. Talk to yourself the way you would talk to your best friend. Be gentle, compassionate, and patient with yourself. There is no right way to get through this, only your way.

Most importantly, I've learned that returning to living is possible rather than remaining a patient. Slowly, I have disconnected from the websites and support groups that were so crucial during treatment. I am healing.

Now, where each day used to be about cancer, it is not anymore. It is about working out, seeing friends, and using my brain again. I am finding my way back to a life centered on living, not just surviving.

What Carries You Through

Cancer reshapes your friendships. Some people disappear, some surprise you, and some become lifelines. What I learned first was that I had to be my own best friend. I had to quiet the mean girl voice in my head and ask her to take a back seat.

At the same time, I craved normalcy. I kept circling back to the same plea in my diary: take me out to lunch, distract me, let me feel like myself again.

That's where Talli came in. She sent me near-daily texts—simple check-ins, nothing elaborate. Sometimes she even pulled me into a silly game of virtual mini-golf. Her steady presence reminded me I still mattered, that I wasn't only a woman with cancer.

Meanwhile, Gus was carrying so much at home, all while I was in chemo. And then, in the middle of it, we had to say goodbye to Dakota.

The weight of those losses piled up, but the steadiness of one friend—and the unshakable grace of Gus—made it bearable. In the end, it wasn't a crowd or grand gestures that carried me. It was the kindness of one friend, the strength of one partner, and the reminder to befriend myself.

Resilience isn't always about doing more. Sometimes it's about recognizing what carries you through—one small act of kindness, repeated again and again.

Chapter 10: Living Forward

After surgery and before radiation treatments began, I was declared **cancer-free**. Even though part of the tumor had still been alive after 12 rounds of chemo, my medical team believed they had removed all of it. My sentinel lymph nodes were clear—a huge relief, especially after remembering how much time the ultrasound technician had spent scanning my armpit back in February. This meant I didn't have to lose additional lymph nodes, and my risk of lymphedema, a lifelong concern for many breast cancer survivors, was almost zero.

Even though radiation was over, my HER2-positive status meant my treatment wasn't entirely behind me. I still needed Kadcyla, a targeted therapy designed to ensure no lingering cancer cells could grow in my body.

What follows are a few diary entries from this phase of recovery. As I started feeling better—as I was mostly recovered from radiation—I didn't write as much. I didn't need to keep people updated on every step. Instead, I focused on something that felt both foreign and familiar: getting back to *living*.

Some challenges remained. The chemo brain fog lingered, making it harder to find words as quickly as before. My sister assured me it would improve with time. She was right.

One thing that never changed was music. Music has always been a massive part of my life, and concerts have been a way to connect, especially with my daughter, Julia, and my husband, Gus. Julia and I have been to 60 shows together. We share a love of singer-songwriters and are always seeking out new artists who pass through Portland. Concerts became more than just events for us; they were milestones, reminders that life wasn't just about survival, it was about love and joy.

Day 193: Kadcyla Begins

I got here at 7:10 am. I checked in, and the nurse accessed my port and drew lots of tubes of blood for a clotting study. My medical oncologist changed my drug, so I had to have it drip for 90 minutes, and now I must wait another 90 to make sure I don't have a reaction. I got some good napping in the chair.

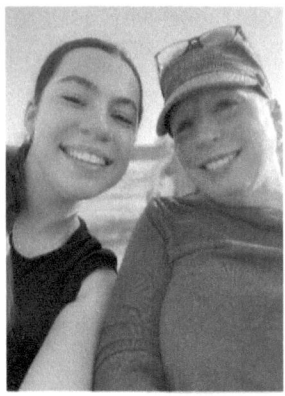

Julia and I went to see Maggie Rogers at Edgefield last night. We had a great time, and Maggie was awesome. Maggie's reminder was great: "If you're not sweating, you're not doing it right." We danced until I couldn't stand up. I'm delighted the temperatures have dropped in Oregon. It was way too hot this week. Cheers, and have a good weekend.

Day 203: Positivity Begins to Return

It has been a little over a week since I finished radiation. I am feeling good!

The burn has gone away. My skin is normal. My boobs are starting to look "normal" to me. I am back at Pilates and taking it easy in the level-one classes. This week, I am going every day. A little sore, but nothing I cannot handle.

I feel almost normal, taking daily Tamoxifen and not experiencing any major symptoms. The chemo fog is lifting. Still struggling for a word here and there. It is nothing compared to what it was a few weeks ago.

We're headed to LA to see Gia and Todd. I'm so excited about visiting them. Then Julia and I leave for Boston to see Mom, my sister, and Patrick. It has been too long.

I am up for anything. Call me if you want to talk, eat, or walk!

Had fun shopping with Sarah and walking around the park with Talli. Loved the phone call from Vicki and my sister Ali.

I appreciate the texts, calls, and support. I'm not sure how much I will type here. Hugs to all.

Day 225: Family Trip & Return to Weightlifting

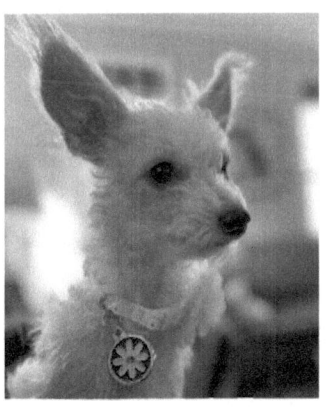

I had a wonderful trip to Boston, where I saw my mom, sister, stepdad, and stepbrother. It was really lovely. I brought our new dog, Georgie, along. She is a great traveler. I have more energy each week. I've been going back to Pilates and working out 6 days a week. I'm still taking level 1 and 1.5 classes, taking my time. It's nice to be back, but it's also weird. People I took classes with before are surprised to see me, and I am still uncomfortable telling people about the cancer.

I cleaned out my bra drawer. I shudder to think how much money is in the pile. I found even more after I took the photo. It feels like a milestone moment to say goodbye to underwires. DDD and higher went straight into the pile. I found one C, but it did not fit well. The cups were gaping. I may well be down to a B. Crazy. 3.5 pounds —how many sizes? I am still a little swollen, so I will not invest in expensive bras for a few more months.

I am returning to weightlifting today. I can hardly wait to see Brett and pump some iron. I am hoping it helps strengthen my bones after all the drugs put me into full-blown osteoporosis.

Wishing you all the best. I would love to grab lunch or chat on FaceTime anytime. Hugs.

I discuss rebuilding strength and protecting bone health after treatment in Chapter 11.

That was the last entry I posted in 2023. Since then, I've finished Kadcyla, had my port removed, and started bone-building infusions with Zometa. My scans in both 2023 and December 2024 came back clean—a relief every time. Those milestones marked the end of the public part of my journey. What followed was quieter and harder to describe: learning how to move forward when the daily battle was suddenly over.

Chapter 11: Rejoining the Living

Day 356: Scanxiety

It's been a while since I've posted. Tomorrow is my first mammogram since the diagnostic that led to my biopsy—almost exactly a year ago. I also have a Kadcyla infusion and an echocardiogram this week, so my anxiety is running high. Early this morning, as I tried to let Georgie out to pee, I smashed my pinky toe on a chair. It's broken and throbbing, which feels about right for the week ahead.

I feel pretty good most days. The daily Tamoxifen makes my joints stiff, but otherwise I'm tolerating the meds. Pilates, weightlifting, and walking Georgie two miles a day keep me moving and grounded. I'm also beginning part-time work again, helping Portland Community College with curriculum design for students interested in tech careers. It feels good to be teaching again.

I'm holding on to the hope that tomorrow's mammogram will be boring and unremarkable. Still, the "scanxiety" is real. Any unusual pain or symptom pulls me back into that familiar fear of: what if it's back?

I've come to accept that this is part of my life now. Any minor symptom, any unusual pain, will always bring that lingering feeling of "what if?" But I remind myself: I've made it through before, and if I have to, I will again.

Rejoining the living – that's a dramatic way to describe what happens after treatment ends. You're no longer driving to the hospital daily or weekly. There are no more infusions or radiation sessions. It's a bit disconcerting. I was lucky that my radiation oncologist, Dr. Lee, was upfront about this transition. On two separate occasions, she told me how hard this next stage can be for many patients.

Dr. Lee explained it this way: for months, I was actively fighting cancer—getting chemo, undressing, going to radiation, getting dressed again, seeing specialists, and visiting the hospital so often I could probably drive there with my eyes shut. (Not really, but you get the idea.) I was in a routine, battling the disease every day. And then, suddenly, it was over. No more treatments. No more weekly checkups. And no daily reminders from medical professionals reassuring me that I was on track.

It was time to move on and get back to living. The challenge, of course, is figuring out what that means. How do you stop obsessing over the next test or whether you're still cancer-free? How do you let yourself live without fear?

My Advice: Have a Plan

Understand what "rejoining the living" means to you. Hopefully, you've maintained relationships and kept your mind engaged during treatment. Here are some things to consider:

- **Work:** Will you return to work? Can you ease back into it? Perhaps start with 10 hours a week, then gradually increase the hours.
- **Healthy Habits:** How will you stay on track with eating well and exercising? For me, it's about consistency. After experiencing a pulmonary embolism, I'm determined to keep my blood flowing and my lungs strong.

- **Social Connections:** How will you nurture your friendships and relationships? Staying connected to others is vital for emotional and mental well-being.

What Worked for Me

I approached my return to "normal" life methodically. Here are a few things that helped me:

Social Routines

I set up regular dinners with my friend Carrie. Once a month, we go out to eat. We don't drink alcohol anymore—she's been incredibly supportive of my need to protect my liver, which went through hell processing chemo drugs in 2023. I still have a drink a few times a year, but nothing like before. Make sure your friends are genuinely invested in your health and recovery. You may also look around and realize that people you thought were your friends were only friends when you were healthy. They may be so afraid of getting sick (as if cancer is contagious) that they have drifted away. That's okay. There is a season for friendships. Those friends won't be the ones who walk into the next season of your life with you. *You'll also hear from Shelby in Chapter 14, where she shares how her friendships and expectations shifted after her diagnosis.*

Pilates and Fitness

Pilates has been my anchor. It keeps me limber, warms up my body early in the morning, and helps me handle my day with energy. After eight years, I'm still not bored, because every class is different, thanks to the instructors' creativity.

Working out with my trainer, Brett, has also been a transformative experience. He focuses on bone strength and healthy aging. We've added exercises like Farmer's Carries (carrying 75% of your body weight in two hands for 1 minute) to load my bones and help rebuild them. You start lighter and progressively overload until you reach the target weight. Studies show that weight training is the best way to combat osteoporosis. I've even started wearing a 16-pound weighted vest while walking, which is within guidelines and about 10% of my body weight.

I also prioritize functional fitness: being able to sit on the floor and get back up without using my hands is a skill I practice regularly. Aging with grace, strength, and mobility is always at the top of my annual goals. Losing weight in the process has been very encouraging. Since I am postmenopausal, that has been a struggle. As soon as Brett had me counting macros and eating five small meals rather than two or three larger ones, the weight started to come off.

Friendships

I'll admit I need to work on this one. Pursuing my master's degree has taken up much of my time, but I do make an effort to stay connected. For example, I meet Vicki once a month for side-by-side foot massages, which I always look forward to. I take regular walks with Talli and her dog, Roxy. I'm working on establishing unique routines with other friends because human interaction and socialization are essential for thriving in this next phase of life.

Personal Growth and Volunteering

Going back to school has been incredibly rewarding, and volunteering has also helped me re-enter the world with purpose. Both experiences have given me a sense of progress and connection.

Moving forward is all about striking a balance: staying active, nurturing relationships, prioritizing health, and pursuing personal growth. Figure out what "living" looks like and take it one step at a time.

Chapter 12: Living with the Unknown

But even as life began to feel more balanced—returning to work, moving my body again, reconnecting with friends—the unknown was always there in the background. What if it comes back? Why did I survive when others didn't? These questions became the quiet companions of survivorship. They don't show up in the treatment plan, but they're as real as any scar or side effect. This chapter is about naming those feelings—fear of recurrence and survivor's guilt—and learning how to live fully, even with uncertainty close at hand.

Dealing with the Fear of Recurrence

Waiting for diagnostic tests can feel like staring into the unknown. For me, it brought back the same fears I had faced when I was first diagnosed. I never felt the cancer in my breast. It was found via a mammogram. None of the doctors or specialists who examined me could feel it either. It was too small.

Nearly two years have passed since that diagnostic mammogram, so when I found a lump in my breast I could actually feel in November of 2024, my mind immediately raced to worst-case scenarios.

It could be a fatty deposit. It could be a cyst.

I hoped it was either or.

But there I was again, back in that place of uncertainty.

I called my doctor the day after I found it, and they quickly scheduled a mammogram and ultrasound. Then, the waiting began.

This time, I handled it better. I leaned on advice from my grandmother, Ruthie: *"Don't borrow trouble."* She was right—there was no need to panic when I didn't have answers yet. I kept my fears contained, sharing the situation only with my sister (a fellow cancer survivor) and my husband. I knew I'd bring more people into the circle if there was something to share.

I've come to accept that this is part of my life now. Anytime something feels off or unusual—whether I'm not feeling 100% or notice a change—I know I'll have to get it checked so I can rule out cancer. It's a constant undercurrent, but I've developed more resilience since 2023. I'm stronger now, and I face these tests head-on.

That doesn't mean I never feel nervous or cry while waiting. I remind myself that, if a recurrence is caught early enough, it's treatable. I hold on to that hope, and I trust my doctors.

In the end, the tests revealed good news: I was cleared for another year.

The lump turned out to be necrotic fatty tissue, a leftover from my breast reduction. It might never be reabsorbed. It could calcify. But it isn't dangerous. It isn't cancer.

Survivor's Guilt—the Unspoken Weight of Making It Through

Survivor's guilt is rarely talked about, but it's something that lingers. Why did I make it through cancer when others didn't? Why do I get more time when my dad doesn't? How am I now older than he was when he died?

The guilt hits in unexpected ways—when I hear about someone else's recurrence, when I see another obituary, or when I remember friends who didn't make it. I lost my neighbor to pancreatic cancer a few years ago. She found love late in life, adopted two beautiful children, and died before she could see them grow up. Grief and guilt are intertwined; learning to live with both is part of finding your way through. Any time I see a small plane go down on the news, I grieve for the family and friends left behind, especially if the cause is not immediately apparent. Living without knowing why someone died is its own kind of loss. *You'll see different perspectives on this in Section Three, where other women share how they've carried survivor's guilt in their own lives.*

Carrying survivor's guilt while still in treatment created a strange tension: I was mourning others while fighting to finish my own treatment, knowing that I would survive. The calendar became my anchor, marking each step toward the end of treatment. And it was time to move on.

Moving On

What I've shared so far is deeply personal—my lens on cancer, loss, and renewal. But as anyone who's faced breast cancer knows, no two stories are alike. The type of diagnosis, the treatment plan, the support system, even the timing in life—all of it shapes how the journey unfolds.

That's why this book isn't just my voice. In Section Three, you'll hear from other women who generously opened their lives to share their experiences. Their stories differ from mine, but are threaded with the same themes of fear, strength, frustration, and hope. Together, they remind us that while every cancer journey is unique, we are not alone.

SECTION THREE
Other Voices

My story is only one version of what it means to face breast cancer. In this section, you'll hear from five women whose lives took very different turns—and yet their strength, struggles, and wisdom echo familiar truths. You'll also hear from my husband, Gus, who walked beside me through all of it. These voices remind us: no one has to face this alone.

The Power of Shared Experience

Facing a cancer diagnosis is a profoundly personal and life-altering experience. No two journeys are the same—every diagnosis, treatment path, and recovery process is shaped by unique factors, from the type of cancer and medical approach to personal support systems and individual resilience. And yet, amid this deeply personal battle, one truth remains: we should not have to walk this road alone.

As we've seen, breast cancer affects one in eight women in their lifetime, a staggering statistic. Yet, when it happens to you, it doesn't feel common—it feels like the ground has been pulled out from under you. You find yourself searching for guidance, for a map through the chaos, and for someone who understands what it's like to stand in this terrifying place.

That's when I called Erin. I knew she had faced cancer a few years before me; when I was diagnosed, I reached out to her, seeking wisdom, comfort, and someone who simply "got it." Later, after I had made my way through the most challenging parts of treatment, Shelby and Aurora were also diagnosed, and this time, they reached out to me. I met Gail through her sister, who reached out to me for advice and support. Vivian is friends with a couple who work out at the gym with my trainer, Brett. Our shared experiences created an unexpected sisterhood—one built not just on living forward but on the deep, unspoken understanding of what it means to hear the words *"You have cancer"* and the countless ways that reality reshapes your life.

Each of our journeys was different. Cancer is never a one-size-fits-all experience. The choices we made, the treatments we endured, and the emotions we wrestled with were uniquely ours. And yet, through our differences, we found a common thread: the power of women supporting women.

The stories in this chapter are personal reflections from these five remarkable women, who have generously shared their thoughts, challenges, and lessons learned. Their experiences may resonate deeply with you, or they may not. That's the beauty of personal storytelling—each journey is unique, and there is wisdom in every story. Some of what they share may feel familiar, and some may feel foreign. What matters most is that these reflections serve as a reminder that no one walks this path alone.

Whether you are reading this as someone newly diagnosed, a friend or family member offering support, or simply as a reminder to schedule your mammogram, I hope these words provide insight, comfort, and encouragement. There is no perfect way to face cancer, but there is beauty in sharing what we've learned and passing that strength forward.

Chapter 13: Erin's Story

Navigating Treatment During a Pandemic and Finding Unexpected Resilience

Erin and I met years ago when our eldest daughters practiced the same sport. While we sat on the sidelines, we'd chat about family, work, and life. Erin was one of the first people I knew who ran a nonprofit's social media page, and I admired the calm, steady way she approached both work and life. When I began my own cancer journey, her presence reassured me.

I asked her what helped her most during diagnosis and treatment. Here's what she shared:

What helped you the most during your diagnosis and treatment?

Two months before my diagnosis, my aunt found a lump, had it removed, and did 16 treatments of radiation. My treatments were different, but we compared notes frequently. In both cases, it was not hereditary. We are the "lucky" ones to be included in the one-in-eight scenario. Being able to call her to vent was pretty cool because she could relate. If you don't have a person to vent to, find one.

Were there any unexpected challenges or moments of hope that stood out?

My diagnosis was in August of 2020, during COVID-19. The whole world was shut down. Everyone was isolated at home, and it felt dangerous to socialize. As a private person, I didn't want to share my story on social media; it was out of the question. Talking about it on Facebook with people I went to kindergarten with didn't feel right. I told people that

I spoke to daily via text or my co-workers on Zoom. Since I wasn't seeing friends in person, I didn't tell many people. The people who did know had never been through it. That was hard but also ok; they just listened a lot. I went to almost all of my appointments alone. People checking in on me afterward was therapeutic.

I asked a lot of questions during appointments. I leaned on the healthcare workers. That's another story; nurses have my heart. Doctors know many things. Nurses know how to manage side effects (and there are a ton of them), and they provide something I can't describe.

I also found Breast Friends, a non-profit that walks breast cancer patients through the process. I felt comfortable asking the group questions on Facebook. And when I didn't want to ask about something, there was a search box that would search for my specific topic. Chances are, if I thought about it at 2 am—and I did—the answer was there. I also attended Zoom meetings with newly diagnosed women and another meeting with women who had various degrees of "problems," looking for support. The later Zoom meetings put me in check; my pity party ended with a hard stop. "What, you've only had one boob for 2 years?" My problem seemed so silly.

What advice would you give to someone newly diagnosed or their loved ones?

There are numerous steps, tests, doctors' opinions, procedures, and paths to follow. Don't get excited or scared when you are on step #1. And if they offer you an antidepressant and sleeping pills, TAKE THEM home! You might need them later, even if you don't need them right now.

How has your perspective on life changed since your diagnosis?

One time, I was running down several flights of stairs in the hospital parking garage because the elevator was taking too long. I turned a corner and almost ran into a homeless man; it scared me. He called me a bitch. Without even thinking, I said, "I have cancer; you can't scare me." This really isn't a perspective on life, but when I think of that afternoon, I feel an emotion I've never had before: I can do this. My whole life, I always thought everything new was scary, but it turns out I can do hard things, which I didn't know before.

Chapter 14: Shelby's Story

Discovering Self-Compassion and Challenging Expectations

Shelby and I worked at the same company for several years, even in the same group at times. I loved her "can-do" attitude and warm, welcoming smile. Every encounter left me energized and excited for what we might accomplish together. When she was diagnosed after me, we spent many hours chatting as she found her footing. Just as Erin had once shared a thoughtful bag of goodies with me, I was able to pass along a similar bag to Shelby. She shares her story below.

What helped you most during your diagnosis and treatment?

For me, it was the wonderful circle of supportive family and friends who made themselves available in every way. Some were sounding boards where I could talk through my worries and irritations. Others shared their own experiences and the helpful tools they used to deal with the side effects of chemo, anxiety around appointments, and dealing with insensitive people. The loving care shown to me was the most edifying, helping me to remember that I wasn't alone in the process.

Were there any unexpected challenges or moments of hope that stood out?

My challenges were related to my self-perception. I feel like my awareness has expanded to 360 degrees, compared to the 180 degrees of everyday life. I was so sick from the chemo, and I was very mad at myself for not being stronger. I realized that I expect so much from myself. My self-talk drove my distress. Thoughts like, *'I shouldn't be sad; I need to be positive; I'm stronger than this; I shouldn't be so angry.'*

I also realized how toxic my closest friend was and how, all these years, I had been suffering mistreatment to be a 'perfect' friend in her eyes. It shattered me, but also strengthened me to be honest with myself. To be for myself, who I try to be for others. I realized that my value of kindness should be applied to myself. Would I expect a friend to be stronger, not sad, and more positive? Of course not. I would embrace them and say, *'I'm here for you. I will help you. I accept you.'* I wouldn't judge or criticize them.

I started allowing myself to experience my emotions instead of beating myself up about them. I began to love and prioritize myself, just as I try to do for others. I had to express myself to that longtime friend, and it felt like a huge weight of resentment had lifted from me. I'm at the tail end of treatment now and feel amazing! I am stronger now because of this cancer recovery journey. I can truly love myself and others more authentically now because of this process.

What advice would you give to someone newly diagnosed or their loved ones?

Find your circle of supportive loved ones or community members. Be kind to yourself as you deal with the overwhelming emotions that will come. Treat yourself to whatever you need to have moments of joy in your daily existence. Maybe that's petting an animal, hanging out with little children, watching comedians on TV, eating your favorite treat, staring out the window, and appreciating the trees, birds, and squirrels. It's taking a moment wherever you can to get out of the dread, the anger, the fear—and bring in a small measure of joy.

Mindfulness plays a big part in my life. I don't say that I have the C word because I feel like that's taking ownership of something I don't want. I use the term *'Cancer Recovery Process'* when chatting with folks to keep a positive spin on it in my subconscious.

Chapter 15: Aurora's Story

Finding Strength in Setting Boundaries

Aurora (not her real name) and I first met at work back in 2010. She's a brilliant woman who loves the intersection of math and people—using data to improve both the work environment and employee skills. I admire her strength and forthright manner, and I've always seen her as a mentor. When she was diagnosed after me, our roles shifted. For the first time, I was the one offering support. She later shared with me what helped her most and what she learned along the way.

What helped you most during your diagnosis and treatment?

The most helpful thing was not telling most of my family— kids, parents, and siblings. I had plenty of non-family people I love, including my partner, who were wonderfully supportive. Sharing my diagnosis only with those who did not feel a personal stake and could support me without making me responsible for their messy emotions was actually really helpful. I feel guilty about not telling my parents and kids, which made for a few awkward moments. Still, it was a relief not to have to manage anyone else's emotions while mine were heightened.

Were there any unexpected challenges or moments of hope that stood out?

The biggest challenge was how my experience both strengthened and damaged my faith in the medical profession. I was amazed by what medical science could do, but frustrated by how often I felt misled. The assurances meant to keep me calm often proved false, leaving me feeling betrayed. However, my partner was an incredible source of strength, and the women I knew who had walked this path before were a true gift. Their empathy and zest for life were my guiding light.

I also found Buddhist ideas about suffering and non-attachment far more helpful than the idea that "everything happens for a reason." That shift in perspective gave me peace.

What advice would you give to someone newly diagnosed or their loved ones?

Figure out what support looks like for you. You do not owe anyone anything here. *Ring Theory*—supporting in and dumping out—is a lifesaver for managing stress and emotions. Remember, science is amazing, and we are so much better at finding and treating this now. Trust the process, but stay informed about what's best for your specific situation.

How has your perspective on life changed since your diagnosis?

My job was eliminated about a month after I shared my diagnosis at work. Whether it was related or not, it compelled me to confront some difficult emotional truths. Work had always been my coping mechanism, and losing that identity while dealing with a health crisis was destabilizing. At the same time, it created space for me to reevaluate how I live my life. I am trying to create more room for other identities and live with more intention. This health challenge has been a good nudge to do that.

Chapter 16: Gail's Story

Taking Control and Advocating for Yourself

About a year after I completed treatment, another colleague from my former workplace reached out. Her sister, Gail, had been diagnosed with aggressive breast cancer. Gail had already done extensive research and was actively exploring her treatment options. She had a few questions for me, and I was glad to offer support. Gail took a very intentional approach to her care, and she shares her insights below.

I'm an n =1. In research terms, that means I'm just one data point. I am one of the eight women who will be diagnosed with breast cancer in their lifetime. Specifically, I belong to the 10–15% of women whose breast cancer is triple negative. My story isn't finished yet, but I've learned critical lessons about taking control and advocating for myself to ensure the best possible outcomes.

What helped you most during your diagnosis and treatment?

Movement was crucial. Having an established cardio and strength routine before my diagnosis was something I was determined to maintain. Even when tired or achy, I committed to some form of daily movement, whether short walks, stationary biking, or gym workouts. Nutrition and hydration were equally important. A protein-rich diet and fermented foods helped support my muscle mass, gut health, and overall recovery. Staying well-hydrated with electrolytes significantly improved my well-being, especially after chemo treatments.

Were there any unexpected challenges or moments of hope that stood out?

Tracking my symptoms, weight, blood pressure, and temperature daily allowed me to anticipate difficult days and manage side effects proactively. An unexpected challenge was the intense bone pain after white cell booster injections, but advocating persistently with my healthcare team led to solutions and significantly improved my experience. Embracing rest without guilt became a healing tool, providing unexpected comfort and promoting recovery.

What advice would you give someone newly diagnosed or their loved ones?

Be proactive about your care. Keep moving, nourish your body, stay hydrated, track your symptoms diligently, and advocate strongly for your needs. Allow yourself the grace to rest deeply. Accept support from loved ones and remember to extend compassion and understanding to yourself throughout your journey.

How has your perspective on life changed since your diagnosis?

My diagnosis and treatment taught me the importance of advocating for myself and not suffering silently. It deepened my appreciation for the support from family and friends, recognizing their crucial role in my emotional and physical recovery. Most importantly, it reinforced the value of rest and listening to my body's needs, transforming my approach to self-care and resilience.

Chapter 17: Vivian's Story

Embracing Gratitude and Faith

Vivian and I met through friends at the gym where I lift weights three times a week. They encouraged me to reach out to see how I might support her and answer questions. Vivian chose to cold-cap—something I didn't do because I couldn't face the headaches from freezing my scalp—and she was able to retain most of her hair. Her story is below.

Diagnosis

I was 41 when I was diagnosed with Stage 2 IDC, ER/PR+ HER2-negative cancer. I scheduled an appointment and saw my primary care doctor in August 2024. My doctor said that she was 99% certain the lump I was feeling on my left breast was just a fibrous cyst, which are common, and would most likely go away. Although I was excited to hear how certain she was that it was nothing to worry about, I had a feeling I needed further confirmation than a "touch and visual" exam. I requested a mammogram, as I was nearly 41 and hadn't had one yet. My doctor advised us to monitor it and revisit in a few months. She ran blood work and came back with low iron. I started taking iron, and it did make me feel better; however, I still didn't feel right. My partner often asked me about getting the lump checked. Since it was constantly on both of our minds, I called and requested to schedule a mammogram for peace of mind. My appointment for the mammogram and ultrasound was on 11/8/24. That day, my world turned upside down. The doctor told me I had breast cancer, but wanted to do a biopsy to confirm. My life has not been the same since.

What helped you the most during your diagnosis and treatment?

What has helped me the most is staying positive through the journey and the multitude of steps involved in beating this ugly monster. Don't get me wrong, I have had moments of anger, disbelief, sadness, and heartache. The highs and lows of being a healthy, positive, and active person, to now being a new woman with the diagnosis, has been overwhelming. I have stayed strong in my faith, reminding myself that God is with me and he will get me through it.

I am grateful to have an incredible boyfriend who has been through every single step of the way with me; keeping me positive, being present at all my appointments, holding my hand through each step, wiping each of my tears, loving me even when my body was changing, reassuring me that everything would be ok, and he was there for it all.

My kids (14 & 17) mean the world to me. Having my kids made things so much more difficult to have cancer, but having them has also made it so much easier to fight cancer. I want to live a long life so I can love them and witness them as they grow into amazing adults. I struggled letting my kids know about my diagnosis, and did not tell them for months, until I had more information, knew the plan, and had more strength to tell them. They have been so supportive and helpful.

My amazing friends and family, who have been there for me through it all. I did not tell many people at first, but I got more and more comfortable as I grew stronger and told more family and friends. At first, it was overwhelming having too many people checking on me, not because they were checking on me, but because I was constantly reminded that I was sick. In my mind, I was trying to make it go away ("I can't be one of 8").

My medical team has been incredible in helping me through diagnosis and treatment. Listening to all my concerns must have sounded like a broken record, but I made sure to ask everything I could. They listened and provided all the answers so I could make proper decisions tailored to my specific cancer and circumstances. All the doctors and their teams, as well as the social workers, have been outstanding in providing information and resources, and helping me navigate through all the steps and challenges.

Cancer survivors whom I was able to reach out to and ask questions that other people couldn't understand. A few friends and friends of friends have not only answered questions but also just listened when I needed to vent, or held me when all I needed was to cry. There are also a couple of Facebook groups that are very helpful.

Were there any unexpected challenges or moments of hope that stood out?

Yes, so many! On this journey, I have tried hard to find silver linings in every challenge.

Challenge 1: I had to do four TC chemo treatments (a common combination of Taxotere and Cytoxan) after initially being told I wouldn't need chemo but only surgery and radiation. Chemo was such a scary word – the next scary "C" word I had to hear. It made me upset, then really mad to know that I would lose my hair. I am so grateful for the nurse who helped me and brought up Cold Capping. Exploring the option of cold capping to keep my hair gave me so much hope. I was so afraid of going bald because of my kids. They knew I was sick, but I didn't want them to *see* that I was sick. Through patience and a lot of work done by my boyfriend, I was able to keep some of my hair.

Challenge 2: Genetic testing was offered since my aunt had breast cancer. I have the BRCA2 gene, which has made my journey somewhat more understandable, but also more challenging. More testing and a change in my surgery and therapy options came into play. I am grateful for such advanced discoveries and medicine tailored to those of us who were gifted this gene.

Challenge 3: In addition to the BRCA2 gene mutation, I also have a prothrombin gene mutation, which causes my blood to clot more than normal. This, too, has been a learning experience for me and my medical team. They have narrowed down what the best options are for me, and I am hopeful it will be. On top of radiation, I will have my ovaries removed soon, followed by hormone therapy.

What advice would you give to someone newly diagnosed or their loved ones?

Stay positive even though it's hard. Do fun things and have events on the calendar to look forward to. DON'T cancel life because of cancer. Don't let it scare you to the point of missing out on fun things. Obviously, there will be times when you don't feel well, and you should stay home and rest. Your doctors will support you in living a safe and healthy way.

Accept help when loved ones offer it. It is hard to ask for help, but on this journey, it is so much easier to navigate with people's help. Even if it's small things or just dinners dropped off. You are not alone!

Lean on other survivors, but don't compare your journey to anyone else's: it's yours and yours only. Even though a lot of things are out of your control, you still get to make choices that fit you and no one else. Be your own advocate and ask as many questions as it takes to understand. If it doesn't feel right to decide right away, wait. Your medical team will understand and will help you when the time and the options are right.

Allow yourself to feel all the emotions that come with being diagnosed and experiencing the long journey. Cry when you feel like you need to. Some days are good; enjoy them. Some days are rough; learn from them and don't let them take you down for too long. Above all, love this new version of yourself!

How has your perspective on life changed since your diagnosis?

Absolutely. When we are young, we feel like life is forever. I never thought I would be sick this young. There is no doubt that cancer has no preference and doesn't discriminate. It can happen to anyone, at any age, any time. I always thought that being kind to everyone was important because we don't know what battle they are fighting. Now, more than ever, I am trying to practice kindness not only toward others but also toward myself. This world is ugly, but I believe that life is still beautiful. No matter what our challenges are, there is so much to live for; it is worth the fight.

My medical team has been incredible in helping me through diagnosis and treatment. Listening to all my concerns must have sounded like a broken record, but I made sure to ask everything I could. They listened and provided all the answers so I could make proper decisions tailored to my specific cancer and circumstances. All the doctors and their teams, as well as the social workers, have been outstanding in providing information and resources, and helping me navigate through all the steps and challenges.

Cancer survivors whom I was able to reach out to and ask questions that other people couldn't understand. A few friends and friends of friends have not only answered questions but also just listened when I needed to vent, or held me when all I needed was to cry. There are also a couple of Facebook groups that are very helpful.

Were there any unexpected challenges or moments of hope that stood out?

Yes, so many! On this journey, I have tried hard to find silver linings in every challenge.

Challenge 1: I had to do four TC chemo treatments (a common combination of Taxotere and Cytoxan) after initially being told I wouldn't need chemo but only surgery and radiation. Chemo was such a scary word – the next scary "C" word I had to hear. It made me upset, then really mad to know that I would lose my hair. I am so grateful for the nurse who helped me and brought up Cold Capping. Exploring the option of cold capping to keep my hair gave me so much hope. I was so afraid of going bald because of my kids. They knew I was sick, but I didn't want them to *see* that I was sick. Through patience and a lot of work done by my boyfriend, I was able to keep some of my hair.

Challenge 2: Genetic testing was offered since my aunt had breast cancer. I have the BRCA2 gene, which has made my journey somewhat more understandable, but also more challenging. More testing and a change in my surgery and therapy options came into play. I am grateful for such advanced discoveries and medicine tailored to those of us who were gifted this gene.

Challenge 3: In addition to the BRCA2 gene mutation, I also have a prothrombin gene mutation, which causes my blood to clot more than normal. This, too, has been a learning experience for me and my medical team. They have narrowed down what the best options are for me, and I am hopeful it will be. On top of radiation, I will have my ovaries removed soon, followed by hormone therapy.

What advice would you give to someone newly diagnosed or their loved ones?

Stay positive even though it's hard. Do fun things and have events on the calendar to look forward to. DON'T cancel life because of cancer. Don't let it scare you to the point of missing out on fun things. Obviously, there will be times when you don't feel well, and you should stay home and rest. Your doctors will support you in living a safe and healthy way.

Accept help when loved ones offer it. It is hard to ask for help, but on this journey, it is so much easier to navigate with people's help. Even if it's small things or just dinners dropped off. You are not alone!

Lean on other survivors, but don't compare your journey to anyone else's: it's yours and yours only. Even though a lot of things are out of your control, you still get to make choices that fit you and no one else. Be your own advocate and ask as many questions as it takes to understand. If it doesn't feel right to decide right away, wait. Your medical team will understand and will help you when the time and the options are right.

Allow yourself to feel all the emotions that come with being diagnosed and experiencing the long journey. Cry when you

Chapter 18: A Note from Gus

A Husband's Journey

This section wouldn't be complete without hearing from my closest companion on my cancer journey, my husband, Gus. I know how lucky I am to have had a partner who showed up with support, compassion, humor, and love. He's a quiet and reserved person, in contrast to me, who is more animated and expressive. I was honored when he answered my questions and shared the following responses.

The First Text

When I first read Vikki's text on the plane about her diagnosis, I felt dread. Terror. Not knowing the complete diagnosis, what would come next, and how I would deal with the situation.

I felt what I felt. I didn't feel the need to process it. Or if I did, I would just process it in my own way at my own pace, while I worked to solve the problems at hand.

The Hardest Part

The hardest part was watching her struggle with the challenge, watching the disease and the treatment take so much vitality out of her and not leaving her with the energy to do any of the things that define who she is.

I didn't find anything that I had to do to support her to be burdensome. I tried to find ways to be helpful and supportive, and doing these things helped me stay centered and focused on the future.

I compartmentalized. It was the only way I could stay sane. Focus on the most urgent problem or need at hand, take care of that, and then move on to the next thing, doing whatever

I could think of that would be helpful or caring in the moment.

Trying to Empathize

I tried to be as empathetic and supportive as possible. I have not gone through any major illness or any course of treatment like Vikki experienced, so I didn't have any prior frame of reference.

I tried as best I could to empathize and give her what I thought she needed in the moment, without making any judgments or assumptions, knowing I couldn't really understand, in a deep, familiar sense, what she was going through.

I don't look back and wish I had said or done anything differently; only that if there were some way I could've done more, I wish I'd known it in the moment.

Staying Grounded

I focused on Vikki, or on my mom when she needed it. Not on me or anything else. Just figure out what needs to be done, how to be helpful in the moment, and just do it. Moment by moment, day by day.

I should probably have had more outlets. Practicing mindfulness and having an exercise routine helped. I really appreciated other folks helping out—providing dinners, taking Vikki to some appointments, and just being helpful. That was a big morale booster.

What I Learned

We can get through even the hardest of times if we stick together and rely on love. What an absolute shit year 2023 was. There was a lot of heartbreak and challenges. Taking it one day at a time, and always together, is the way to get through the worst of times.

And I know that Vikki did everything in her power not to put a burden on me, even though she didn't have to. If she asked me for something, I knew it was because she absolutely needed it and couldn't do it herself. I knew I had to be attentive to her needs because she wouldn't necessarily tell me when she needed something. I knew I couldn't be complacent.

Advice for Other Caregivers

Focus on your partner. Try to put yourself in their shoes in the moment and imagine what would be appreciated most to get through the next hour or the next day.

Find whatever hacks you can to make things easier for you—order meal kits to help with the daily hassle of meal preparation, accept any help friends or family offer, and try to keep as many normal activities going as possible. Continue engaging with family and friends and adhere to daily routines as much as possible, making adjustments as necessary. Don't sweat the small or unimportant stuff. Save your energy for the big, important things. Decide what's essential; whatever isn't, put it in a box and don't worry about it.

The Bad and the Good

The bad moments will come, and they may be really bad. The time when Vikki was first adjusting to chemo was harrowing. She had aches in her bones so bad that it completely immobilized her, and there was nothing I could do to alleviate her pain. Coupled with the terrible outbreak on her skin, so bad she had to go on steroids—that was the worst.

I was terrified. Is this what we will have to endure for the next year? What if she couldn't tolerate this? What then? Not being able to do more killed me. Having such a supportive and engaged medical team to get us through that was critical.

The good part was that the chemo killed her face spiders[13] and all but eliminated her rosacea. The other good part was confirming that we could get through the worst life can throw at us together without coming apart.

Love and Attention

You can get through it together with love and compassion. In addition to providing all the support and more your partner needs, be attentive and try to anticipate their needs. Your partner may not tell you to avoid putting a burden on you, or they might not even know what they need in the moment. From your perspective, you may see what will be helpful.

Stay attentive. Stay kind and compassionate. Ensure you put in place a structure or plan to get through it, day by day.

We hope our experiences give you strength and practical tools for your journey. You are not alone.

Moving On

Stories have the power to make us feel seen; to remind us we belong to a community of survivors and caregivers who understand. But sometimes, when you're in the middle of treatment or supporting someone you love, you also need

---

"Face spiders' is Gus's nickname for **Demodex mites**—tiny organisms that live in facial hair follicles and can worsen rosacea. During chemo, my skin erupted with painful pustules, but afterward my rosacea disappeared for two years before roaring back. That's when my dermatologist prescribed **Rovis Gel**, which has been a game-changer. Gus still laughs at the nickname—and if you google them, you'll see why.".